细胞自稳机制
与癌症特异性堵酸门
治疗

Autostabilisis
and Blocking-acid-gate
Therapy Specific to Cancer

国 前◎著

郑州大学出版社

图书在版编目(CIP)数据

细胞自稳机制与癌症特异性堵酸门治疗／国前著. — 郑州：郑州大学出版社，2021.11

ISBN 978-7-5645-7505-2

Ⅰ.①细… Ⅱ.①国… Ⅲ.①癌-细胞-诊疗 Ⅳ.①R73

中国版本图书馆 CIP 数据核字(2020)第 222076 号

细胞自稳机制与癌症特异性堵酸门治疗

XIBAO ZIWEN JIZHI YU AIZHENG TEYIXING DUSUANMEN ZHILIAO

策划编辑	李龙传		封面设计	曾耀东
责任编辑	薛 晗		版式设计	凌 青
责任校对	刘 莉		责任监制	凌 青　李瑞卿

出版发行	郑州大学出版社有限公司		地　址	郑州市大学路 40 号(450052)
出 版 人	孙保营		网　址	http://www.zzup.cn
经　销	全国新华书店		发行电话	0371-66966070
印　刷	河南大美印刷有限公司			
开　本	787 mm×1 092 mm　1/16			
印　张	7		字　数	177 千字
版　次	2021 年 11 月第 1 版		印　次	2021 年 11 月第 1 次印刷

书　号	ISBN 978-7-5645-7505-2		定　价	49.00 元

前　言

　　癌症是严重威胁人类健康和致人死亡的重大疾病。多少年来,人类为了癌症的预防和治疗付出了巨大的人力和物力。虽然取得了一些成就,但是癌症在全世界总的发病趋势仍在继续上升,总的死亡率仍位居各种病因之第二。而癌症患者的死亡,90%以上是由于癌细胞的恶性生物学行为——侵袭和转移造成的。这也是癌症难以治疗的根源。那到底是什么原因导致了癌症的转移? 采用什么样的对策可以遏制其恶性生物学行为,并以较少的费用即可对其实施治愈性的医疗措施呢? 如此关键的问题之所以久攻不破,是因为长期以来人们缺乏对癌细胞产生恶性生物学行为的关键原理的认识,因而导致了缺乏理论指导的针对癌细胞侵袭性生长与远处转移的特异性治疗措施。针对上述攻克癌症必须面临的关键问题,本书从基础的细胞分子生物学到临床的医学实践,通过全系统的层面,对癌细胞恶性生物学行为产生的关键机制——如何通过抗圆缩凋亡和致死性微管介导的基因组不稳定作用从而逃避细胞生长的自稳机制予以了阐明。本书所提出并阐明的细胞生长自稳机制是高级多细胞生物的"生命咽喉"式立命之本。这一概念揭示:无论什么样的癌细胞(各种实体癌和血液癌,如白血病)通过无论什么样的基因改变,若要想获得癌细胞的恶性生物学行为表型,其遗传学和(或)表观遗传学变异的结果必须满足限制三磷酸鸟苷产出通路这一独特性代谢条件,只有这样才能够逃避圆缩凋亡与致死性的微管介导的基因组不稳定的"刹车"作用,进而使癌细胞可以摆脱细胞自稳机制的生长限控、演化出其侵袭与转移的恶性生物学行为。本书根据所揭示的这一自然规律性概念为基础形成的指导性治疗理论,对癌症临床治疗方案的具体实施做了进一步的阐述。基于癌细胞获得恶性生物学行为的这一独特规律,作者设计和建立了一种针对其代谢特点的"堵酸门"治疗方案。该方案除了能够特异性地杀灭具有恶性生物学行为的癌细胞、预防和阻止癌细胞的侵袭性生长和远处转移、杀灭休眠的癌细胞预防癌症的复发、重塑异质性癌的组织结构从而为手术创建多重窗口期之外,还具有相较于传统癌症疗法毒副作用小、维持患者的生活质量高、治疗途径简单以及治疗费用低廉等特点。另外,由于细胞自稳机制对高级多细胞生物的存在起着"生命咽喉"式的立命作用,即没有细胞自稳机制就不会有高级多细胞生物,因此由微管介导的基因组不稳定和圆缩凋亡构筑的细胞自稳系统机制自然地铸成了生物医学诸多重要科学谜题的实质与核心。正是由于此概念对于高级多细胞生物生命规律的基础性、普适性与重要性,遵循这一纲领性概念为线索的研究,可使得长期困扰着科学家的许多重要谜题迎刃而解。对此,本书在第二部分对以此概念为核心机制的系列重要生物医学谜题进行了揭示,例如,近1个世纪的生物医学谜题——以其发现者、诺贝尔生理学或医学奖得主 Otto Heinrich Warburg 名字命名的瓦伯格效应的生物学功能与临床意义是什么? 为什么现有的技术手段难以克服严重的实体干细胞治疗安全性瓶颈问题,即无法避免干细胞治疗带来的大规模基因突变的致病风险,包括致癌性;为什么半个多世纪以来,被誉为生物学顶梁柱的海弗里克极限所显示的人的正常细胞只能经历50~60次群体倍增寿命极限的著名经典假说只是反映细胞在体外人为条件下非生理性圆缩而产生的基因组不稳定性以及大规模基因突变的典型命运,并不能作为任何指标反映人体正常细胞的生理性生命极限,也不能用此推断和说明人的寿命;端粒长度为什么不能用作支持海弗里克极限的理论基础? 癌细胞为什么会休眠与复发? 癌症患者为什么会出现恶液质? 外伤为什么会导致青少年骨肉瘤? 再有,为什么有了"垃圾"DNA才会有了高级多细胞生物? 此阐述从理论上解答了《科学》杂志提出的125个重大科学前沿问题中的"基因组中的'垃圾'有何作用"的谜题,为癌症治疗方案的建立奠定了指导性理论基础;等等。本书破解性阐明的诸多谜题不仅关乎人们对癌症与相关疾病本质的认识、奠定上述癌症治疗方案的理论基础,而且对人们认识自然科学规律、扩充科学知识、对治疗和预防相关疾病以及进行相应的科学研究实践都具有重要的指导意义。

Foreword

Cancer is a major disease that seriously threatens human health and causes death. Over the years, human beings have devoted tremendous manpower and material resources to the prevention and treatment of cancer. However, the overall incidence of cancer in the world still continues to rise, and the mortality rate ranks second among all human diseases. Why is cancer so difficult to cure? The main reason is the lack of essential understanding of the malignant biological behavior, invasive growth and distant metastasis of cancer. The lack of understanding of the key principles of generating malignant biological behavior leads to the lack of theoretical guidance for the specific treatment of invasive growth and distant metastasis. Invasive growth and distant metastasis of cancer are the causes of death in more than 90% of cancer patients. Unfortunately, the existing cancer treatment methods have no specific therapeutic effects on the invasive growth and distant metastasis. To solve this problem, two questions are naturally raised. One is what is the mechanism of enabling cancer cells to invade and metastasize? Another is what kind of specific and low-cost methods against the malignant biological behaviors can be used to cure cancer?

This book systematically answered the two questions based on the author's discovered machinery —"autostabilisis" (Greek, auto means "self", stabilisis, "stand"; all that means "maintenance of the stability of cellular growth"), which plays the "life throat" in cell-growth control of advanced multicellular living beings. The concept of autostabilisis reveals that the results of whatever genetic and/or epigenetic variations have to fulfill the unique metabolic condition of restricting guanosine triphosphate (GTP) production pathway if the malignant-biological-behavior phenotype of cancer cells is to be obtained, regardless of any kind of cancer cells (solid cancers and hematological cancers — leukemia). Only in this way can cancer cells escape the "braking" effect of circompactosis (Latin, circ means "round", com, "intensive", pact, "fasten", and sis, "state of death"; all that means "cell death caused by the effect of cell rounding") and lethal microtubules-induced genomic instability (MIGI), thus enabling cancer cells to evade the growth restriction of autostabilisis and evolve their malignant biological behaviors of invasion and metastasis. Based on the unique rule that cancer cells acquire their malignant biological behaviors, the author has designed and established a "blocking-acid-gate (BAG)" therapeutic regimen aiming at cancer cells' metabolic characteristics. It can specifically kill cancer cells with malignant biological behaviors, prevent and block their invasive growth and distant metastasis, kill dormant cancer cells to prevent their recurrence, and remodel the tissue structure of heterogeneous cancers into a growth-pattern similar to benign tumors, thus creating a multiple window period for curative surgery. Compared with traditional cancer therapy, this regimen not only has the characteristics of less toxicity and side effects, but also has the characteristics of maintaining patients'life in higher quality, and making treatment simple and in low cost. In addition, autostabilisis plays a "life throat" role in the existence of advanced multicellular living beings, that is, there would be no advanced multicellular living beings without autostabilisis, so the autostabilic machinery constructed by MIGI and circompactosis naturally cast the essence and core of many important biological and medical puzzles.

Following the concept of autostabilisis as a clue, researches can solve many important puzzles that have plagued scientists for a long time, such as: what are the biological functions and clinical significance of the Warburg effect? Why can't current technology guarantee the safety of solid stem cell therapy? What is all that "junk" DNA doing in our genome? Why do cancer cells go dormant and relapsed? Why does cancer patient appear cachexia? Is somatic cell cloning safe? Why can't the Hayflick limit reflect the physiological life span of normal cells? Why can't telomere length be used as a theoretical basis for supporting Hayflick limit? Why does trauma cause osteosarcoma in adolescents? And so on. To clarify these puzzles is not only related to people's understanding of the nature of cancer and related diseases, laying the theoretical foundation of the above cancer therapeutic regimen, but also has important guiding significance for expanding scientific knowledge and carrying out corresponding scientific research practice.

For simplicity, the detailed discussion in the book is divided into two chapters. The first chapter describes the principle and strategy of specific BAG therapy for cancer metastasis, and the second chapter expounds many scientific puzzles based on autostabilisis, circompactosis and MIGI.

目　录

第一章

▶治疗原理与方案

一 高级多细胞生物的细胞存活的关键机制

　　生命的本质是存活和繁衍,无论人体正常细胞还是癌细胞均是如此。细胞则是构成生命体的最基本单位。对于高级多细胞生物来讲,细胞要达到存活和繁衍这两项生命目标,必须完成两项相应的至关重要的细胞与分子生物学活动。其一,为了存活,细胞就要建立与维持以各种蛋白质为基础的生物功能体系,而该体系的核心蛋白质的产生离不开其关键基本环节 RNA 的转录。其二,细胞要繁衍增殖,即由一个细胞变为两个细胞,就要进行细胞物质材料的倍增;其中,承载生命密码的遗传物质 DNA 的合成复制是至关重要的;完成这一过程,需要经历一个被人为定义的细胞生长与分裂的周期,即所谓的细胞周期,该周期被分为 DNA 合成前期($G_{0/1}$ 期)、DNA 合成期(S 期)、DNA 合成后期(G_2 期)和有丝分裂期(M 期)。那么对应于 RNA 转录和 DNA 复制最为关键的限制因素或者说是高级多细胞生物的细胞存活的关键机制又是什么呢? 答案就是细胞核的大小。

　　大家都知道,自然界的万物存在与活动都需要空间。奠定人体细胞存活基础的各种生物分子间的生化反应更是如此。细胞虽然属于微观级别,但细胞内的各种反应绝非是杂乱无章。DNA 是人体细胞中的巨分子,一个人体细胞的 DNA 分子长度可达两米。如此长的 DNA 分子只有被高度压缩后,才能被包装在仅有数微米大小的细胞核中。并且,只有 DNA 分子经过缠绕压缩形成染色体,才能够使得复制好的 DNA 在有丝分裂(M 期)时被分配给两个子代细胞。但是,处于染色体状态的 DNA 在空间上自然地限制了其 RNA 的转录和 DNA 的复制。然而子代细胞要开始新的细胞周期生命活动,不仅需要将 DNA 由紧密压缩的染色体变为结构疏松的染色质,而且还要解螺旋,并将双链 DNA 分开成为单链 DNA。所有这一切必须在细胞核的空间变得足够大时才能进行。问题来了,体细胞是怎样增大其细胞核的呢? 答案是通过贴附而完成的铺展。

二 癌细胞恶性生物学行为的细胞生物学基础

当细胞刚结束 M 期分裂成为两个子细胞时，细胞呈圆形，且并未与其周围的细胞外基质以及其他邻近细胞建立相关的连接，DNA 也呈压缩状态。随着子细胞的贴附、铺展以及与其他邻近细胞连接的建立，细胞核开始变大，DNA 也由染色体变为染色质，细胞开始生长，随即开始了下一个细胞周期。这是在生理状态下，正常细胞生长增殖的情况。而癌细胞又是怎样生长增殖的呢？回答这个问题，首先要从众所周知的癌症置人于死亡的一个重要原因就是侵袭和转移这样一条线索来探讨。为什么癌症会发生侵袭和转移呢？这还得从癌细胞的细胞生物学改变说起。从事肿瘤临床，尤其是学习过脱落细胞学和病理学的人都知道，癌细胞在诊断上的最主要特点之一是细胞核的增大，这一特点适合于确定所有类型的癌细胞恶性程度的诊断，包括实体瘤性癌细胞和血液癌细胞，即白血病细胞。为什么？前边我们讲过，只有细胞核的增大才能使 RNA 的转录和 DNA 的复制得以进行，细胞也才能够存活和增殖，而癌细胞的细胞核增大则与其恶性生物学行为构成了密切的因果关系。那么癌细胞的核增大机制与正常细胞的核增大机制有什么不同吗？要搞清这个机制，我们须更进一步到细胞分子生物学来找答案。

自然界的任何物质要发生形态的改变都离不开力的作用，细胞核要改变大小也不例外。人体细胞中存在着两种主要的力，这两种力构成了决定细胞核大小的关键因素。由于这两种力的相互制衡，才维持了人体细胞的有序生活与自身稳定，这就是高级多细胞生物存活的"生命咽喉"，本书称其为细胞自稳。那这两种力是什么呢？这就是由微管产生的压缩力和由肌动蛋白产生的牵张力。对于正常细胞来说，当细胞贴附于细胞外基质铺展的时候，由肌动蛋白纤维产生的牵张力对抗了由微管产生的压缩力，使细胞核得以生理性增大，以满足 RNA 的转录和 DNA 复制的要求。此时，二力的相互作用达到一种生理性平衡，从而维持细胞有序的生存和增殖。一旦这种力的平衡关系由于肌动蛋白赖以产生牵张力的细胞黏附连接的破坏而丧失，则界面张力和由微管产生的压缩力即会成为优势，细胞随即发生圆缩，正常细胞的细胞核也自然地被剧烈压缩变小（图 1-1）。

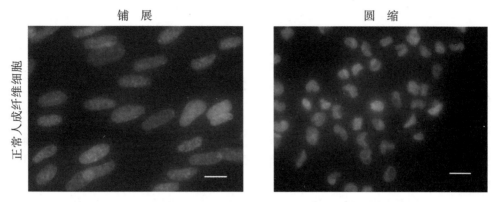

图1-1 正常细胞铺展与圆缩时细胞核大小

　　但对于癌细胞来说,其不受控制的存活、生长、侵袭和转移特性要求其必须在不依赖贴附、铺展于细胞外基质的情况下,仍然能够有别于正常细胞,维持足够大的细胞核(图1-2)。这一关键因素就是铸成癌细胞臭名昭著的侵袭性生长和远处转移恶性生物学行为的基础。循着细胞核大小决定细胞生死这条线索无疑可以找到答案。并且通过对此问题的深入剖析,自然可以揭示出用于指导癌症治疗的细胞分子生物学特性。接下来,还是把癌细胞远处转移作为切入点,进行相关的深入阐释。

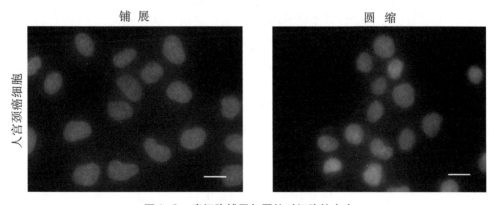

图1-2 癌细胞铺展与圆缩时细胞核大小

三　高级多细胞生物的细胞自稳核心机制——圆缩凋亡

既然是远处转移,顾名思义,癌细胞就要离开原发的部位,通过体内的循环系统到达远处的转移器官。于是,最重要的问题就出现了,为什么脱离原位的癌细胞在循环系统非贴附的状态下能够存活? 要回答这个问题,就要提出一个概念,即圆缩凋亡(circompactosis)(该词源自拉丁语,circ 意为圆形,com 为剧烈,pact 为紧缩,sis 为一种死亡状态)。此概念是指,由于各种原因,细胞失去在生理状态下维持其细胞核大小的牵张力,从而使得细胞发生圆缩,并且,细胞核在微管产生的压缩力的作用下缩小,进而导致细胞死亡的事件。之所以要提出这样一个概念,是因为之前人们观察到一种现象,即正常细胞和一些不具有转移性的肿瘤细胞在脱离其附着的细胞外基质和相邻的细胞后,即发生一种特殊方式的细胞死亡,被称之为"失巢凋亡"。虽然,对"失巢凋亡"的抗拒是造成癌细胞远处转移的前提条件,已被医学界公认。然而,或许正是因为这一概念的定义是基于"失巢",才使得之后对于其机制的探讨几乎都是围绕着所谓的"信号转导"而展开。因为,看起来似乎"失巢"就断开了细胞间以及细胞与细胞外基质间的所谓信号分子的链接,于是就发生了信号转导变化的问题;但也正是由于这种先入为主的惯性思维,才限制了我们对于与此密切关联的生物现象的本质认识;使得之前人们不能够解释为什么细胞只是发生了圆缩,但并未失去与细胞外基质或细胞的连接,即并未"失巢",却仍然要发生凋亡这一谜题。然而,这是一个不能回避的原则问题,澄清这一迷题的背后机制,对于探讨癌症治疗问题意义重大,所以在此要提出"圆缩凋亡"这一具有双重意义的概念,它既可以从细胞与组织病理学层面上揭示其现象,又可以从细胞和分子生物学层面上对其发生机制予以阐明。

在上面谈到的认为"失巢凋亡"是"信号转导"发挥控制作用的观点中,以整合素为关键分子构成的黏着斑激酶(focal adhesion kinase,FAK)信号通路成为了"失巢凋亡"诸多信号通路观点的核心代表。然而,无论何种"信号转导"的阐述,都无法对与之密切相关的凋亡进程中细胞存活的关键问题予以解释。

依据"信号转导"的观点,细胞"失巢",凋亡信号才予以触发,细胞也才会发生凋亡,但事实并非如此。当单个与细胞外基质或邻近细胞贴附的正常细胞在"不失巢"的情况下,只要发生圆缩,若不能够得到进一步铺展,则细胞仍难逃凋亡的命运。不仅如此,传统认为的信号转导机制对于"失巢凋亡"还有如下无法做出解释的问题。第一,既然"失巢凋亡"是由于细胞脱离贴附触发了凋亡信号,为什么正常细胞在脱离贴附后,经历相当长的一段时间(数小时)后,再行贴附、铺展,细胞并不发生凋亡? 换句话说,脱离贴附所触发的凋亡信号作用何在? 再退一步说,假如"失巢凋亡"是可逆的,那可逆的信号通路是什么？第二，如果细胞脱离与细胞外基质的连接即会触发凋亡信号的产生，为什么正常细胞形成悬浮球，并不与细胞外基质发生接触？虽然已"失巢"却也不会发生凋亡？究竟细胞的基质贴附与细胞间的连接在"失巢凋亡"中的作用是什么？第三，细胞脱离贴附多长时间，再行贴附铺展，可避免凋亡发生？为什么（这里一再强调铺展，因为单纯贴附是不能避免凋亡的）？要回答这些问题，还是要回到 RNA 转录的问题上来。细胞的生理功能维持，离不开细胞内的各种生物化学反应，而各种生物化学反应则有赖于各种相关蛋白质的参与。因此，"失巢凋亡"的机制问题也就显而易见了。由于细胞发生了圆缩，细胞核就会被压缩，RNA 就不能完成生理功能性的转录，没有了 RNA 的这种转录，也就不可能有相应的蛋白质翻译。虽然人体内的各种蛋白质半衰期长短不一，从几十秒到几百天不等。但短寿蛋白通常对于代谢起着关键的调节作用。所以，mRNA 的这种转录阻滞和蛋白质的无从翻译，以及已转录的 mRNA 和已翻译的蛋白质寿命的终结所造成的生化反应紊乱与停滞，造成了"失巢凋亡"呈现出的"延时性"死亡与脱落时限性的可逆"再生"模式与现象。因此，提出"圆缩凋亡"的概念，不仅可以反映细胞核大小与细胞死亡的规律、涵盖其发生机制，而且还可以由此得到关键性的提示，即癌细胞圆缩时细胞核增大（相较于正常细胞而言）的维持不仅对癌症转移意义重大，而且也是癌细胞侵袭性生长的前提与基础。

四　上皮组织结构与癌细胞生长的关系

人体 90% 以上的恶性肿瘤来源于时时刻刻都在持续生长增殖与更新的上皮组织，所以要阐明癌细胞恶性生物学行为的产生问题，还是要从了解正常上皮的组织结构来探讨。正常上皮细胞具有两个极，一个叫作顶极，另一个叫作基底极。细胞以基底极附着于基底膜上生长与增殖。细胞与细胞之间形成多种连接，包括紧密连接、间隙连接、带状连接、桥粒连接、半桥粒连接等。位于细胞顶端的紧密连接具有阻止大分子物质透过的封闭作用。而细胞的基底面和基底侧面分布着不同的生长因子受体。各种细胞生长所需的生长因子以限控性的方式透过基底膜到达细胞的基底面和基底侧面与其相应的受体结合，从而刺激细胞的增殖。正常细胞在这种组织结构下以一种有序可控的方式生长。而在癌症发生与形成过程中，随着细胞的极性结构消失和基底膜被破坏，使得细胞趋向于变圆、组织结构对生长因子的限控性消失，细胞的生长方式就会变得无序、失控。为了进一步理解上皮组织结构对细胞生长的调控作用，这里还要阐明另一概念——细胞接触抑制。

所谓"接触抑制"是指当正常细胞生长达到汇合时，细胞就会停止生长。而癌细胞则不会发生接触抑制，所以呈现为叠层堆积性生长。为什么？因为正常细胞的增殖依赖于生长因子的作用。前面讲过上皮组织解剖结构的特点，也就是由于正常上皮细胞顶侧面的紧密连接的封闭作用,决定了生长因子的基底侧供给。正常情况下,生长因子不可能从细胞的顶侧面越过紧密连接与位于细胞基底面和基底侧面的生长因子受体结合,也就不能产生刺激细胞增殖分裂的信号作用。作者之前对此曾做过专门的研究。研究结果提示,所谓接触抑制,实际上只是体外细胞培养的一种人为现象,在体内是不存在的。如果把细胞处于接触抑制状态的培养皿底部的非通透性结构做局部改变,使其成为大分子可透过性结构,有趣的现象就出现了。未做透过性改变的部位细胞处于所谓"接触抑制"的静止状态,而改变之处细胞则呈现为活跃的叠层堆积性生长。对于癌细胞来讲,由于其细胞连接结构的破坏和极性的丧失,以及突变产生的生长因子自分泌和(或)生长信号转导相关的激酶异常激活等情况,细胞始终都可处于相应的生长信号通路的激活状态,自然也就不存在接触抑制的现象。总之,由于各种方式的遗传与表观遗传的变异均会导致正常组织结构的改变与癌细胞的圆缩。此时的癌细胞若具备了抗圆缩凋亡的遗传学改变,其恶性表型就会出现(快速生长、低分化、侵袭与远处转移)。而趋向于良性方式生长的恶性肿瘤细胞(依赖于外部的生长信号刺激,生长缓慢、高分化、无侵袭与远处转移)则难逃圆缩凋亡的命运管控。临床上,越是分化差的癌细胞,越趋向于变圆,越易于从癌组织脱落。这种现象恰对应于其臭名昭著的恶性生物学行为——侵袭生长和远处转移。本来,细胞脱落是多细胞生物一种不可避免的生物学事件。而为了维持其自身的稳定,防止原位异常生长以及脱落细胞的异位种植性生长,多细胞高级生物才演化出了圆缩细胞的核压缩所致的圆缩凋亡这样一种自限性与细胞自稳性机制。

那么,除了前面讨论的细胞核压缩所致的 RNA 转录阻滞及其圆缩凋亡之外,核压缩还会对细胞产生什么其他重要的影响吗?答案是肯定的。如果留意观察和思考,大家是不是会发现这样一个问题。正常贴附生长增殖的细胞,只有进入 G_2 期的时候,细胞才开始变圆。接下来,子代细胞一旦进入 G_1 期,又开始贴附生长。但是,在病理状态下(如体内的炎症和肿瘤等),以及体外的人为干预(如细胞培养的传代),处于各细胞周期时相的细胞会被剥离、从细胞外基质脱落和发生圆缩。在 S 期,细胞的双链 DNA 必须随着细胞的铺展、核的增大而解螺旋并分开成为单链。此时若遭遇细胞核的剧烈压缩是否会对细胞的再生长产生重要的影响呢?下面将对此进行探讨。

五 细胞核压缩对 DNA 保护机制的灾难性破坏作用

前面谈过,细胞核的压缩会阻滞 DNA 的合成,然而这只是冰山一角,更令人震惊的是细胞核的压缩会导致细胞基因组构成基础的 DNA 发生器质性的改变,并给细胞造成严重的生物学行为性质改变的遗传后果。因为 DNA 与蛋白质均是生物高分子化合物,所以二者也具有分子构象变化的化学特性。处于 S 期的 DNA 能进行复制的前提是细胞核具有足够的空间,以克服 DNA 碱基黏滞性造成的错误配对结合,从而保证其能够从螺旋状态解旋分离成两条单链 DNA,形成复制叉,再进行 DNA 的半保留复制。这一复制过程是在多种蛋白质组成的复制子的参与下完成的。其中,复制蛋白 A(replication protein A,RPA),作为单链 DNA 结合蛋白,主要起着维持 DNA 双链分离后形成复制叉单链 DNA 的稳定,以防止错误的 DNA 二级结构(包括染色体内和染色体间)发生的关键作用。然而,由于细胞圆缩产生的剧烈细胞核压缩,其结果会导致单链 DNA 与 RPA 的构象发生改变。这是否会影响到二者的结合呢? 若结合受到影响,RPA 就会丧失其保护功能,其后果对于细胞来说将是灾难性的。这种基于分子构象改变而影响二者结合力的假设是否为真,关键有赖于下述的实验检测予以证实。

六　细胞原位电泳技术方法的建立与重要意义

　　既然要检测 RPA 与单链 DNA 的序列非特异性结合是否会受到核压缩导致的构象变化的影响,那么检测就必须建立在维持细胞原本核压缩状态的情况下进行。若一旦检测过程破坏了细胞圆缩形成的细胞核的压缩状态,RPA 与 DNA 的结合就会发生改变,二者在核压缩情况下的结合状态也就不能够得到真实的反应。所以目前以凝胶阻滞试验(即 DNA 迁移率变动试验)、染色体免疫沉淀技术(chromatin immunoprecipitation,ChIP)等为代表,以细胞破碎步骤为样品制备前提的方法(即先需要将细胞破损后,再提取DNA-蛋白样品进行后续的繁杂实验分析),均无法满足在维持细胞核结构压缩的情况下,对单链 DNA 与 RPA 结合状态的检测需要。为了能够在不破坏细胞结构的前提下,检测 DNA 与 RPA 的结合状态,作者研发并建立了一种称之为细胞原位电泳(cell in situ electrophoresis,CISE)的技术方法,原理如图 1-3 所示。由于 DNA 系长链"巨"分子,不能透过经微孔处理的细胞质膜。当 RPA 与 DNA 结合后,虽然对细胞施以电场力,但是,由于其与 DNA 的结合,RPA 仍会被锚定在细胞内部。相反,与 DNA 的结合已发生解离的RPA,则会在电场力的驱动下泳出细胞。经此原位电泳的细胞再通过流式细胞术检测其胞内存留的 RPA,就可以反映 DNA 与 RPA 的结合状态。原理虽然并不复杂,但若建立这样一套完整的技术方法体系却并非易事。原因在于该技术方法的建立是基于一个双因素未知的实验体系:第一,RPA 在细胞核压缩的情况下会发生与已结合的 DNA 进行分离只是一个假设,是否为真,无人知晓。第二,如何对假设进行检验,既没有现成的方法,也没有类似的先例可以参考。举个例子,前人做得既成功又成熟的一项实验,而你用自己的方法却做不出来,毫无疑问,肯定是自己的方法出了问题,只要自己做对了,肯定也能做出来;但若前面没有人做出来过,你自己也做不出来,于是心里就会产生这样的压力:到底能不能做出来、做这件事的理论对还是不对、是理论错了还是方法有问题? 这种双未知因素的研究是很容易造成心理压力的。在这种不知自己的设计思路是否正确、技术条件是否可行、多长时间才能完成、是否确定可以实现的情况下,真是压力巨大。再者,整个检测体系中的数十个参数条件需要摸索、优化,可谓牵一发而动全身。从实验设计到仪器制作,再到获得完美的实验结果,经历了无数次的失败,历时近两年才得以实现。令人欣慰的是实验结果完全支持原先的假设。这项工作的完成,终于搞明白了困扰着作者多少年的系列谜题。为接下来的癌症治疗找到了理论的依据。

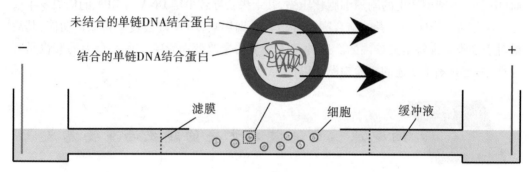

图1-3 细胞原位电泳原理

七 细胞圆缩造成的灾难性基因组不稳定作用

众所周知,在空间高度压缩的细胞核内,存在着大量碱基互补的 DNA 重复序列。由于 RPA 与单链 DNA 结合的解离,单链 DNA 也就丧失了 RPA 为其提供的防止生成错误的二级结构的重要保护作用。同时空间的剧烈压缩,极大地增加了单链 DNA 链内及链间互补碱基序列的可触及性。这就不可避免地会发生染色体内和染色体间的单链 DNA 错配互补结合,从而形成错误的二级结构。虽然细胞内存在着一定的 DNA 修复机制。但是,修复的能力是受到错误程度限制的,否则就不会存在致死性突变的概念。再者,每一个人体细胞内存在着 40 000 ~ 80 000 个 DNA 复制起始点,若没有如此大量的 DNA 复制起始点,细胞就不可能在一个细胞周期中完成 30 多亿个碱基对的庞大 DNA 复制。这也同时意味着,在 DNA 复制期间,一个细胞内的 40 000 ~ 80 000 个复制叉处的 80 000 ~ 160 000 条单链 DNA 在受到 RPA 的保护。一旦细胞遭遇非生理性细胞圆缩导致的核压缩事件,如此大量的单链 DNA 就可能失去 RPA 的保护,其后果注定是灾难性的,要么是导致细胞死亡(致死性基因突变),要么是虽不致死,但造成无法复原性修复的 DNA 损伤(非致死性基因突变,甚至染色体畸变)。

原理相通的事件与概念的发生与存在是自然界的特点和规律。无独有偶,研究进一步发现,端粒保护蛋白 1(protection of telomeres 1,POT1)就是具有类似 RPA 结合特点的另一个可致细胞灾难的因子。POT1 也是一个单链 DNA 结合蛋白,它与其他蛋白一起形成 6 个蛋白的端粒蛋白复合体,在端粒的保护、维持与延长方面起着至关重要的作用。

而端粒是染色体末端的一段保护性 DNA 序列,对保护染色体、维持染色体的正常结构、维护基因组的稳定性方面起着关键性的作用。作者的实验显示,与 RPA 类似,由细胞圆缩造成的细胞核压缩,同样可导致 POT1 与其结合的端粒单链 DNA 的解离。端粒保护蛋白的关键作用之一,就是防止染色体末端的融合与异倍体的形成。因此,细胞圆缩导致的 POT1 与其结合的 DNA 发生解离所造成的端粒失去保护的事件及其 DNA 损伤后果,加之细胞圆缩所致 RPA 与其结合的单链 DNA 解离的后果,二者双重叠加,理论上会产生 1+1>2 的累积效应,这无疑会对于圆缩细胞造成灾难性的 DNA 损伤,且实验结果已证实如此。

总之,正常细胞在圆缩时将产生由微管介导的核压缩效应,包括细胞核压缩导致的 RNA 转录阻滞与圆缩凋亡,以及细胞核压缩导致的 RPA 和 POT1 与其结合的单链 DNA 解离造成的微管介导的基因组不稳定性(microtubule-induced genomic instability,MIGI)。MIGI 的作用直接造成基因变异、染色体畸变、异倍体形成,其后果包括致死性的细胞急性死亡与非急性致死性的细胞衰老。然而,癌细胞为了逃过这多重劫难(其实是机体的一种限控性细胞自稳机制),会通过无论何种形式的基因突变和(或)表观遗传学改变构建一种细胞与分子生物学机制来避免细胞核被压缩的情况发生,从而维持癌细胞在经历圆缩的情况下得以存活,使恶性侵袭性生长和发生远处转移成为可能。至此,又回到了问题的焦点,什么机制使得癌细胞圆缩时仍然能够维持细胞核的增大呢?

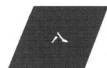

八 癌细胞逃避核压缩性细胞自稳机制

自然界的形变无不是由于力的作用。细胞核的增大也无疑是属于形变的范畴。前面谈过,细胞内存在两种主要影响细胞核形态的力,一种是由肌动蛋白产生的牵张力,另一种是由微管产生的压缩力。当肌动蛋白产生牵张力所必须依赖的细胞与细胞连接的破坏或细胞与细胞外基质贴附力的弱化,以及由于组织正常力的支撑点改变所导致的牵张性消减时,维持生理状态细胞核大小的力的平衡将被破坏。这自然就造成了微管产生的压缩力成为主导作用力,细胞即发生圆缩(circular contraction & compaction,CCC),于是细胞核被剧烈地压缩变小(图 1-1)。

追根溯源,既然压缩力来自于微管,那么微管的改变就应当影响到压缩力的产生。的确如此,当人的正常成纤维细胞经长春新碱(vincristine,VCR;一种抑制微管蛋白组装的药物,已被用作常规工具药)处理后,原本细胞圆缩后出现的细胞核剧烈压缩即可被抑制(图 1-4)。进而,作者又设计了一种细胞悬浮培养实验装置并完成了一项独特的药物实验。将正常人成纤维细胞分为药物处理和对照组,均由贴壁培养转为悬浮培养。药物处理组全程用传统抑制微管组装的抗癌药物长春新碱处理。之后用流式细胞术检测圆缩凋亡。与对照组相比,经长春新碱处理的细胞其圆缩凋亡率显著降低。那么,癌细胞是不是也通过改变微管的组装来控制细胞核的压缩,从而逃避圆缩凋亡的呢? 如果答案是肯定的,会是通过什么样的方式呢? 这还是要从微管的组装机制来分析。

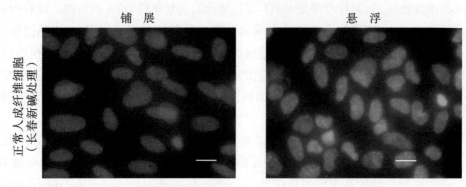

图1-4 长春新碱处理后的正常细胞铺展与悬浮时细胞核大小

微管的组装所必需的两种最重要元素是微管蛋白和三磷酸鸟苷(guanosine triphosphate,GTP)。如果缺乏 GTP 则微管就不能完成适量的组装。若不能满足产生压缩力的微管组装,那癌细胞的细胞核不就可以逃脱细胞圆缩时的被压缩了吗? 如果是这样,癌细胞会通过什么样的方式来减少 GTP 的产生呢?

在生物化学的能量代谢中,有一个核心的产能过程叫三羧酸循环(tricarboxylic acid cycle,TAC)或柠檬酸循环,也被称为 Krebs 循环(以其著名的发现者,1953 年诺贝尔生理或医学奖获得者 Hans Adolf Krebs 的名字命名)。在这个循环中有一个关键步骤,也是唯一直接生成高能磷酸键的反应,即琥珀酰 CoA 在琥珀酰 CoA 合成酶的催化作用下,水解高能硫酯键,与 GDP 磷酸化耦联生成了 GTP。这是正常细胞在氧气充足的生理条件下的代谢产能过程(图1-5)。而癌细胞即使在氧气充足的条件下,也要走另外一条被称为有氧酵解的代谢途径。这一现象是由获得 1931 年诺贝尔生理或医学奖的 Otto Heinrich Warburg 于 1924 年发现的,即著名的瓦伯格效应(Warburg effect)(图1-6)。虽然瓦伯格效应得到了科学界的普遍公认。并根据其发现的这一重要癌症代谢现象研发出了当今世界上最为先进的广谱癌症临床诊断设备——正电子发射断层显像(positron emission tomography,PET)。然而,之前学术界对于瓦伯格效应的背后机制却没有合理的解释。即,为什么癌细胞放着高产能的路(每消耗一分子葡萄糖能产生 36 分子 ATP)不走,却非要走低效(每消耗一分子葡萄糖只能产生 2 分子 ATP)的产能之路呢?

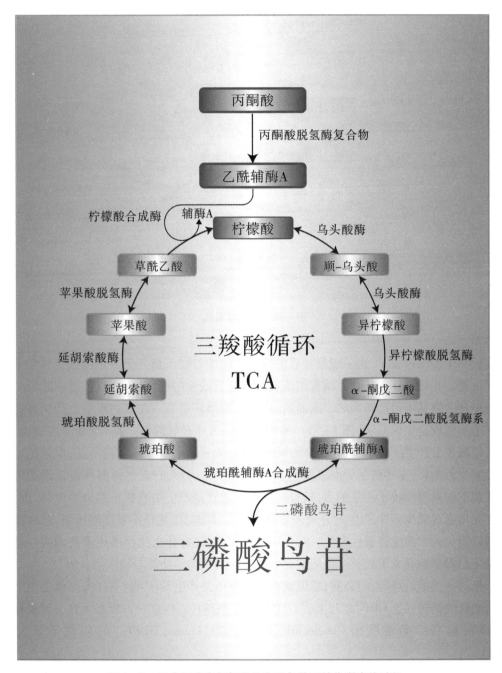

图1-5 正常细胞在氧气充足生理条件下的代谢产能过程

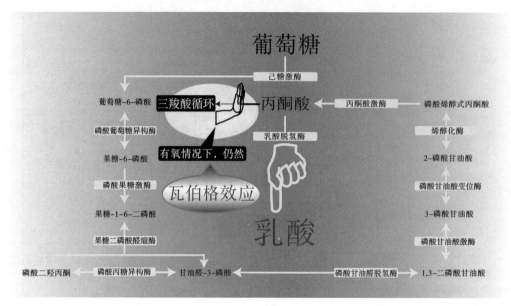

图 1-6　瓦伯格效应

　　近一个世纪过去了,这一现象背后的生物学功能与临床意义仍然是困扰着科学家的不解之谜。是缘分还是巧合? 循着细胞核增大这条线索的探究可以发现,癌细胞躲避三羧酸循环之路是不得已而为之。上面谈过,三羧酸循环中唯一在底物水平上产生高能磷酸键的步骤就是生成 GTP(图 1-5)。癌细胞如果选择有氧酵解之路、避开三羧酸循环,就可以减少 GTP 的产生。由于 GTP 的减少,组装微管的必需原料就会不足,微管的组装就会减少。的确,多年前尽管尚未阐明其生物学意义,但人们观察到多种转化细胞伸展到质膜下的微管相较于正常细胞,只有一半。而微管是产生细胞核压缩力的来源,因此,癌细胞可通过减少 GTP 产生的方式来维持细胞在圆缩时细胞核不被剧烈压缩,从而使细胞得以避免死亡而维持恶性存活。对于生物体来讲,还有什么比存活更重要的吗? 这不就是人们渴望地寻求了近一个世纪的瓦伯格效应的生物学功能与临床意义吗!?

　　探讨到这里,也许人们会问,难道就没有别的通路产生 GTP 吗? 有的,那就是由 ATP 将高能磷酸键转移给 GDP,此乃生成 GTP 的第二条路径。但这一过程必须在一种被称作 Nm23 的核苷二磷酸激酶(nucleotide diphosphate kinase, NDPK)的催化下来完成(图 1-7)。

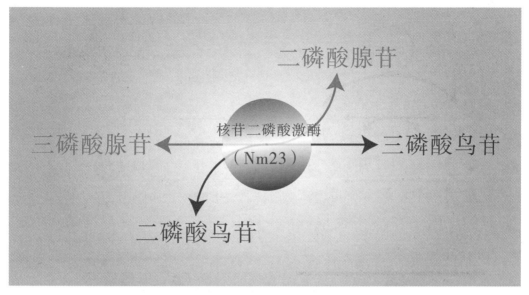

图 1-7 Nm23 的酶促作用

令人惊奇的是,*Nm23* 是人们确立的第一个癌细胞转移抑制基因。Nm23 的表达与多种癌症的转移以及病人的存活呈负相关。虽然其在生物化学中的酶促反应作用早已明确。然而,在细胞与分子生物学层面上,为什么 Nm23 的高表达能够抑制癌细胞转移的机制仍然是个近 30 年的未解之迷。如今根据细胞核压缩所致细胞灾难性后果的研究不难发现,癌细胞 Nm23 的低表达,是从另一条路径上遏制了 GTP 的产出(图 1-8)。它与癌细胞的有氧酵解一起加入到了阻滞微管组装的细胞生物学级联过程,从源头上,减少或消除了由微管产生的力对细胞核的剧烈压缩作用,为癌细胞的抗细胞自稳机制性存活与转移奠定了细胞分子生物学基础。实际上,根据生物化学酶促反应的原理,癌细胞有氧酵解所致的 ATP 减少(氧化磷酸化 36 ATP∶有氧酵解 2 ATP)也在一定程度上可以减少GTP 的产量。

总之,GTP 减少的代谢改变,作为关键性因素,铸成了癌细胞臭名昭著的恶性生物学行为通过抗圆缩凋亡与致死性 MIGI 而得以存活,进而使侵袭性生长与远处播散转移成为可能(图 1-9)。

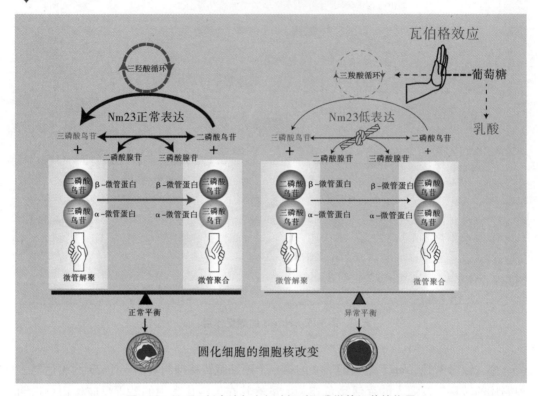

图1-8　Nm23低表达与有氧酵解对阻滞微管组装的作用

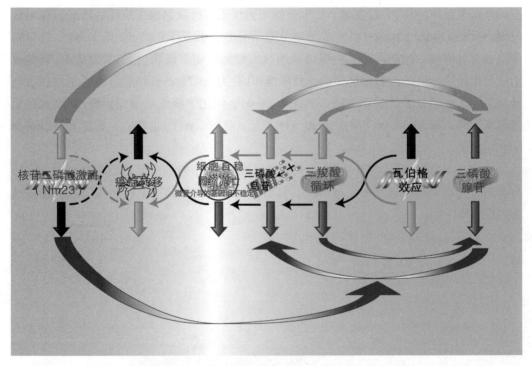

图1-9　GTP、Nm23、瓦伯格效应、ATP与癌细胞恶性生物学行为的关系

九 破解癌细胞逃避细胞自稳机制的谜题对于癌症治疗的理论指导意义

从以上的探讨可以知道,对于高级多细胞生物来讲,圆缩凋亡和致死性 MIGI 是生物体为维护其遗传与生存而进化出的重要的自身稳定性机制。而癌细胞要能够进行快速侵袭性生长和发生远处转移,就必须避免圆缩凋亡和致死性 MIGI 的发生。癌细胞之所以选择有氧酵解通路正是为了逃避圆缩凋亡和致死性 MIGI 而进化出的一种最易行、高效和安全的代谢模式。因为只有这样才可以大规模地限制能够产生核压缩力的微管组装,同时又不至于影响构成纺锤体正常结构的微管形成。换句话说,也就是这样通过 GTP 量的调节,只会影响到微管的大范围产量,而不会引起微管质的改变。否则,对一个细胞来讲,一旦组装的微管发生遗传性的器质性结构改变,严重影响到有丝分裂,其偶发后果要么是致死性的,要么会导致基因组不稳定,但频发的终极遗传后果将是致命性的。既然 GTP 与微管组装减少所致的细胞核免于压缩这一途径是极具恶性生物学行为的癌细胞赖以存活的关键咽喉通路,若能够针对其细胞分子生物学特点,设法发现其"阿喀琉斯之踵",并实施致命的干预性措施,就能够本着"打蛇打七寸"的原则,实现找准命穴一剑封喉的效果,致癌细胞于死地。那么,癌细胞的死穴究竟在哪儿呢? 我们还是要循着细胞核压缩的这条线索来寻找。

癌细胞为了避开三羧酸循环的 GTP 产生途径,不得不选择另外的歧途即有氧酵解。但是有氧酵解的一个重要特点,是会产生大量的乳酸。瓦伯格效应揭示癌细胞糖酵解数量高达正常代谢细胞的 200 倍(此乃现代临床应用的重要高科技癌症发现与转移诊断技术 PET-CT 原始发明的依据)。这就意味着癌细胞不得不采用相应水平的措施把细胞内的乳酸向细胞外排出。因为人体细胞内的各种生化反应对于代谢的酸碱平衡有着十分苛刻的生理性要求(接近中性)。乳酸堆积的后果是非常严重的。临床经验告诉人们,乳酸性酸中毒的结果是致命性的。而癌细胞的乳酸外排既可以避免其胞内酸中毒,同时又为其存活和侵袭扩散与转移创造了条件。因为它破坏了癌细胞周围正常组织和细胞的微环境,造成正常细胞的死亡和细胞外基质的破坏与降解。根据癌细胞这种代谢特点,我们何不将计就计,利用其破坏正常组织的手段来一个"以其人之道,还治其人之身"、针对其"阿喀琉斯之踵"的逆袭呢?

中国传说,古代有一种神兽,名为貔貅。其神奇之处在于,被玉皇大帝封了后门儿("肛门"),即有嘴无肛,可以只进不出。而癌细胞却不是玉皇大帝的貔貅,整日里吞噬大量人体营养,制造并外排大量乳酸来祸害正常人体。我们若能堵住其外排乳酸的"肛门",让大量乳酸潴留在癌细胞自己的胞内,岂不就可以达到既杀死癌细胞,又不伤及正常组织的特异性治疗效果吗? 并且,面对乳酸的大量产生,哪怕是少量的封堵也会导致癌细胞内部乳酸的严重蓄积。正像对于汹涌而来的大洪水,泄洪渠道稍有不畅,便会造成洪水的泛滥。而同样的泄洪条件,对于涓涓细流却无关大局,没有多大影响。那我们采取怎样的措施,才能够实现这一目标呢?

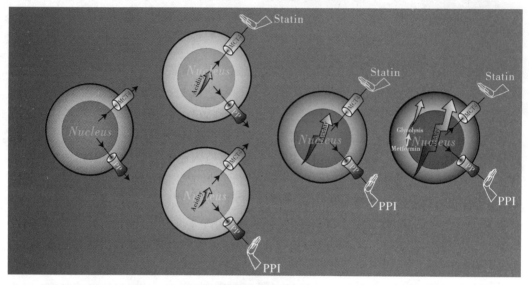

MCT4:单羧酸转运蛋白4;PP:质子泵;Statin:他汀;PPI:质子泵抑制剂;Acidity:酸性;Metformin:二甲双胍;Glycolysis:糖酵解。

图 1-10　堵酸门治疗原理

　　首先要找到癌细胞的后门儿,即乳酸外排的通道。在细胞膜上存在着一个单羧酸转运蛋白(monocarboxylate transporter,MCT)家族。其中的 MCT4 主要负责将大量的由糖酵解产生的乳酸运送到细胞外的作用(图 1-10)。另外,细胞膜上还存在着一种被称为质子泵的物质,可以把细胞内的氢离子泵出细胞外。如果能够阻断维系癌细胞内酸碱平衡的主要通道,就堵住了癌细胞外排大量乳酸的后门儿,从而让癌细胞发生自身酸中毒,给癌细胞造成致命的杀伤。癌细胞的命门儿找到了,接下来的工作是要找封堵剂。大家知道,若要研发一种作为封堵剂的药物,其费用通常是惊人的(几十亿美金),时间是漫长的(通常 20 年左右),且失败的风险巨大(一般在 90%)。感谢大自然的恩赐,让我们在这山穷水尽疑无路的时候,看到了柳暗花明又一村。大家知道,有一类用作降血脂的药物他汀。这种药物有一个最严重的副作用是横纹肌溶解症。为什么?因为横纹肌是人体最重要的运动组织。在无氧运动的时候,横纹肌会因为无氧产能而进行糖酵解,产生大量的乳酸。此时若不能够将这些乳酸通过 MCT4 排出到细胞外,就将造成细胞内乳酸的堆积,接下来的严重后果就自然是横纹肌的溶解性坏死。而他汀类药物恰恰就是 MCT4的抑制剂。所以,只要我们合理地掌握药物的剂量,同时避免不适当的无氧运动和造成正常组织缺氧的事件,并根据癌细胞乳酸产出高于正常组织 2 个数量级(2 orders)(图 1-11)的特点合理用药,就能够特异性地杀死癌细胞而不伤及正常组织(图 1-10)。再者,为防止癌细胞通过质子泵的作用来逃避胞内的酸性封杀,我们可以利用现有的质子泵抑制剂,如奥美拉唑等进行第二重阻滞(图1-10)。还有,在治疗糖尿病方面,有一类药物双胍。双胍类药物最严重的副作用是乳酸酸中毒,这也是双胍类早期药物(苯乙双胍、丁双胍)被停用的原因。目前临床上广泛使用的二甲双胍其乳酸酸中毒的副作用较双胍类早期药物已降低了很多。然而,其仍然具有同样的药理作用。所以,利用其增加乳酸生成的作用就可以进一步提高导致癌细胞酸中毒的胞内酸蓄积水平,构成对癌细胞的助力性杀伤(图1-10)。因为,在合理的药物剂量下产生的乳酸,对于正常细胞的作用只是微乎其微,但对于原本乳酸产出水平较高的癌细胞来讲,无异于是雪上加霜。这也是对癌细胞施加的第三重杀伤力量。再者,血小板在癌细胞的黏附性存活与转移方面起着关键性的作用。为进一步阻断癌细胞的团块性出逃与抱团性存活逃生通道,我们采用应对这一作用的安全药物——阿司匹林、华法林来构筑起置癌细胞于死地的第四重杀手锏。在这四重药物的作用下,具有侵袭性快速生长和远处转移恶性表型的癌细胞就会得到遏制。

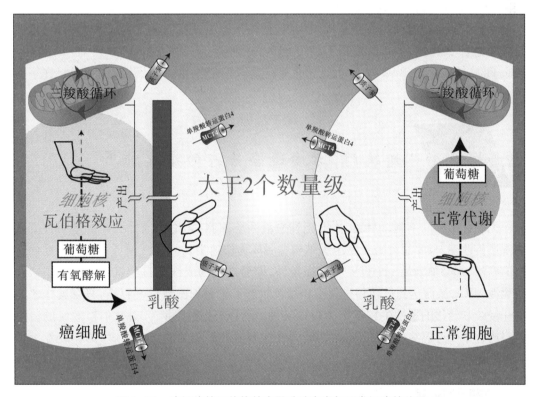

图1-11 癌细胞的瓦伯格效应及乳酸产出与正常细胞的差异

如果癌细胞不走有氧酵解这条路,又会是什么样的结果呢?癌组织是高度异质性的细胞群体。当极具快速侵袭性生长和转移等恶性生物学行为的癌细胞群体被控制和杀灭之后,有些癌组织可能会有残余的、分化较好的、尚未走上有氧酵解通路的癌细胞亚群。这种通过"异质选择"方式存活的癌细胞，只能以近似于正常组织细胞或良性肿瘤的模式生长，并且对放化疗都是耐受的或者说是抗拒的。针对这种情况，我们可以尽可能地通过手术、消融、瘤内注射（机制在后讲）等手段予以斩首式、铲除性治疗。当然，对于难以一次性全部切除的肿瘤，可以采用尽最大可能减少瘤荷的手术措施。然后，再通过上述药物方案治疗，将原先的或后续变异产生的侵袭性癌灶的状态重构成近似良性肿瘤的癌组织与正常组织的边界关系，创建新的手术窗口期，再次施行手术。之所以能够这样做，是基于本药物治疗方案具有控制癌细胞播散转移的关键作用。在此条件下，就可以建立一种全新的手术指征概念，遵循类似于针对良性肿瘤的治愈性手术方案，但要包括转移病灶的切除。因为，其一，此时的癌细胞不以浸润和转移性方式生长；其二，此药物治疗方案可以预防围手术期癌细胞的转移。退一步说，如果此时的癌细胞通过基因变异（如 MIGI 作用）或表观遗传学的途径突破类似良性肿瘤的生长模式，那就只能走向有氧酵解的路径，此药物治疗方案针对的就是这种细胞。否则，发生圆缩的癌细胞若不通过有氧酵解之路试图远处转移，其注定的命运只能是自然地走向衰老和死亡，即使成为漏网之鱼，有了如此天罗地网般的全身性药物加各种手术方案治疗，也会为实施治疗癌症的综合措施赢得时间和奠定基础。当然，任何治疗方式都有其适应证和禁忌证，也就是说无论什么样的治疗方法都不是万能的，这种堵后门使癌细胞酸死的"堵酸门"（blocking-acid-gate，BAG）方法也是如此。有关不适宜采用该方法治疗的情况将在下面进行介绍。

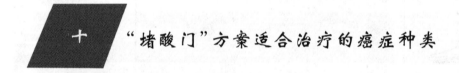

十 "堵酸门"方案适合治疗的癌症种类

无论什么样的细胞，包括实体细胞和血液系统细胞，无论凭借什么样的基因突变或表观遗传改变，只要想突破正常组织结构发展成为快速生长和进入循环系统进行远处转移的癌症，都必须满足一个重要的前提条件，即通过抗构成细胞自稳机制的圆缩凋亡和致死性 MIGI，从而达到在转移过程中和侵袭状态下逃避细胞自稳性存活，只有这样才能够让侵袭和转移的恶性生物学行为得以实现。所以，理论上讲，针对瓦伯格效应的治疗策略适合于所有癌症（包括实体瘤性质的癌症和血液系统的癌症白血病）的侵袭性生长和远处转移。

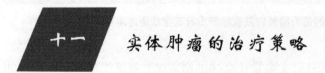

十一 实体肿瘤的治疗策略

手术彻底切除癌组织是目前全世界公认的唯一对实体肿瘤可以达到根除性的治疗

手段。然而,令人遗憾的是很多病人的肿瘤在发现的时候,已经发展到现有手术方法无法彻底切除的阶段;或者癌细胞已发生远处转移,而目前现有的技术手段却对其无法予以检测,即使通过手术对原发灶进行了切除,其亚临床转移灶也会很快发展成为临床转移癌;再或者,由于手术的复杂性与技术的局限性,使得手术操作不可避免地造成癌细胞的扩散;另外,由于肿瘤的恶性生长,已造成了重要器官的弥漫性侵袭受累。在这些情况下,手术的可行性、手术的意义以及手术的效果会受到传统疗效评价的质疑。其质疑的焦点,无疑是手术治疗的局限性。其局限性原由归根结底还是所有恶性肿瘤的万恶之源:侵袭与转移。因侵袭与转移乃癌症难以治疗和致死性的罪魁祸首。而本研究所探讨的系统性治疗方案正是以特异性地针对癌细胞侵袭性生长和远处转移为前提的。本系统方案主要的治疗作用包括:①对癌细胞的代谢呈现为高有氧酵解模式的肿瘤,可予以杀灭;②对适合立即手术的肿瘤,可起到术前预防和术后杀灭残留的高转移性癌细胞的作用,避免手术可能造成的转移;③对不适合立即手术的肿瘤,可先杀灭侵袭性和可能发生远处转移的癌细胞,防止癌细胞远处转移,并将异质性的肿瘤重塑为类似于良性肿瘤生长模式的肿瘤,创造能够施行手术的窗口;④对癌症确诊时,原发灶已发生远处转移,根据现行治疗标准,认为失去手术意义的病人,可先杀灭原发灶侵袭性和可能发生远处转移的癌细胞,防止原发灶癌细胞的远处转移和继发灶癌细胞的再次转移,将原发灶与继发灶异质性的肿瘤重塑为类似于良性肿瘤生长模式的肿瘤,创造具有手术意义的治疗窗口;⑤对术后具有高度复发倾向的病人,可预防性用药,杀灭休眠的癌细胞,防止复发与转移,之所以能够达到这一治疗目标是因为本方案能够特异性地针对休眠癌细胞所具有的有氧酵解模式为主的代谢特点及其从休眠状态被解禁后即可发生远处转移的特性而发挥作用;⑥对脑转移的癌,可采用透过血脑屏障的方案用药,杀灭癌细胞和(或)创造手术窗口;⑦对不以手术为主要治疗手段的肿瘤,可通过用药,杀灭全身性生长的癌细胞(如小细胞癌、大细胞癌等);⑧本治疗方案可缓解由于癌细胞外排乳酸造成的组织乳酸堆积性、非神经损伤性癌痛。

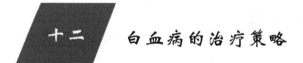

十二　白血病的治疗策略

　　白血病是属于全身性的恶性肿瘤,起源于恶变的造血细胞。白血病的致病特点是,癌变的造血细胞异常增殖,破坏正常的造血组织,使得造血组织丧失其正常的造血功能,并且癌细胞还会侵袭全身重要的脏器,造成贫血、出血、免疫力下降、脏器功能衰竭、脑神经系统损伤等严重的致死性病变。所以,白血病的治疗目标是杀灭白血病细胞,并恢复、重建与维持正常的机体造血功能。

　　虽然目前对于白血病有多种治疗手段(例如放疗、诱导分化、免疫、造血干细胞移植等),但是传统的用药物杀灭白血病细胞的化疗仍然是临床上最基础的重要治疗手段。

特别是对于急性白血病,只有快速有效地控制和杀灭大规模增殖生长的白血病细胞,才能够抢救患者的生命,为后续治疗创造条件,也就是使后续治疗成为可能。然而,传统的化疗及其他杀灭白血病细胞的手段均会产生严重的毒副作用,包括骨髓抑制、肝肾及重要脏器的损伤与功能破坏、免疫功能抑制、严重的消化道反应、感染等;并且周期性的化疗易于使白血病细胞产生耐药性。再者,白血病治疗的费用高昂,无论是对患者及其家庭,还是对社会都是沉重的经济负担。另外,即使对难治性白血病患者付出再高的治疗代价(包括因治疗造成的巨大精神和肉体上的痛苦以及痛不欲生的极其恶劣的生活质量),传统的治疗手段还是对其束手无策,并不能挽救患者的生命。

那么,有没有一种治疗方法能够克服或降低现有治疗手段给白血病患者带来的严重毒副作用并在减轻病人的痛苦、改善与提高病人生活质量的前提下,提高病人的治愈率呢? 这还是要从最基础的白血病发病的细胞分子生物学与组织病理学来探讨。白血病虽然是一种全身性的造血组织病变,并且病变可侵袭全身脏器,但其初始发病并非同时起源于全身造血组织。并且由于血液系统的组织学特点,在发病初始阶段,既无外周血明显变化,又无临床表现,所以很难发现病人的初始病变。而一旦病人以临床症状就诊,则病变往往波及到全身造血组织或其他脏器,病期远非初始病变,所以不会有实体肿瘤的那种"原位癌"概念。而之所以白血病能够发展成为全身造血组织病变并形成全身脏器侵袭的恶性表型,其代谢转变成为有氧酵解为主的模式起到了关键的作用。无论淋巴系还是髓系白血病均是如此。然而,也正是因为这种代谢模式的转变,使之为胞内酸中毒性药物杀死白血病细胞的方法(堵酸门治疗)奠定了治疗基础。并且这种代谢模式的特性自然地赋予了其对应性"堵酸门"方案对癌细胞治疗的特异性;而方案所用的药物又可以克服传统化疗及其他杀灭手段的严重毒副作用;另外其给药途径简单,也为治疗提供了极大的便捷;再者,药物治疗费用的低廉,可为病人、国家减少巨大的经济和社会负担,使千千万万个病人和家庭摆脱治不起白血病的困境。

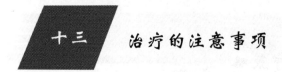

十三 治疗的注意事项

首先,治疗必须严格规范地在专业医生的指导与监控下实施。

任何药物进入人体都要通过相应的组织器官途径,代谢并排出其残余以及有害的代谢产物,否则会造成相应物质的蓄积和中毒。本方案应用的药物也同样需要进行药物代谢,故本方案也有着其严格的适应性病情治疗范围与规则。因此,治疗必须严格规范地在专业医生的指导与监控下实施。另外,除《中国药典》和药物说明书上规定的有关禁忌,下列事项在应用本方案对癌症病人的治疗中尤为重要,必须注意。

无论对于癌症病人还是非癌症病人,机体重要器官的功能衰竭均是造成病人死亡的直接原因。病人一旦发生重要器官的急性功能衰竭,若不能得到有效的治疗改善,病人的病情会急剧恶化,快速导致病人的死亡。而与之相比针对肿瘤的治疗则是一个相对缓慢的过程。所以对于任何原因造成的重要脏器的器质性损伤及其功能不全和衰竭,都要在采取相应的治疗措施,使其基本功能恢复后,才可以应用该方案进行治疗。

重要的脏器损害主要包括:①由化学药物(包括化疗、靶向、镇痛等药物)的毒副作用、放射线损伤、生物治疗(如各种细胞与免疫治疗)的毒副作用引起的肝、肾、心、肺(包括肺纤维化,以及由此导致的低氧血症等)功能不全与衰竭。②由于化学药物毒副作用、放射线损伤和生物治疗造成的重度骨髓抑制,以及癌症转移造成的广泛性骨髓破坏,并由此导致的造血功能丧失。③消化道阻塞(包括食管、胆道、肠道等)。对于此类病人,只有在经过相应的手术(如支架放置、造瘘等)处理,梗阻得到缓解的情况下,才可视病情变化采用该方案酌情治疗。④由化学药物的毒副作用、放射线损伤、生物与免疫治疗的毒副作用及其他因素造成的严重的消化系统损伤与反应。⑤晚期与终末期病人的肿瘤侵袭导致的重要脏器严重器质性破坏,全身多脏器功能衰竭,以及无法进食。

另外,还应注意以下治疗事项:①治疗过程中,避免无氧运动,避免造成全身及局部缺血、缺氧和循环不畅的事件发生。②对未满 10 周岁的儿童以及孕妇,在该方案药物的副作用没有明确之前,不适宜应用。③严格注意奥美拉唑等质子泵抑制剂长期用药可能会产生的副作用,必须合理用药。④理论上讲,二甲双胍与阿司匹林单独使用是把双刃剑,在癌症的不同阶段具有不同的效应,既可以促进癌细胞进化发展,又可以杀死癌细胞,所以要选择合理的复合用药治疗方案以克服单一用药的治疗缺陷并提高疗效。⑤当大量外排乳酸造成癌性疼痛的癌组织被该治疗方案快速杀灭之后,由乳酸引起的癌痛会得到缓解,此时若停止之前大剂量使用的成瘾性止痛药物,则会出现药物撤退性毒品戒断症状。其对应处理需会诊相关学科。

总之,"堵酸门"治疗的特点是杀死以有氧酵解为主要代谢模式的高侵袭与高转移特质的癌细胞;特异性地预防与阻止癌症的初级与次级转移;杀死休眠癌细胞,预防其复发和转移;对于以有氧酵解为主要代谢模式的高侵袭转移性癌细胞被杀灭之后残留的肿瘤,可将其重构为类似于良性的肿瘤,从而创建新的手术窗口期,并可多次施行手术,包括微创介入等联合治疗;对于由癌细胞外排乳酸造成的组织乳酸堆积性、非神经损伤性癌痛可以起到缓解与止痛的治疗效果。

第二章

破解的系列基础生物与临床医学谜题

一 干细胞治疗的安全性瓶颈问题是什么（会基因突变与致癌吗）

随着干细胞的发现，人们对其应用寄予了无限的期盼，希望可以利用干细胞治疗许多疾病。虽然造血干细胞的移植已比较成熟地应用于临床。然而，面对实体干细胞的现实是，胚胎干细胞（embryonic stem cell，ESC）、诱导多能干细胞（induced pluripotent stem cell，iPS cell），以及躯体定向干细胞（committed stem cell，CSC）的应用却非易事。人们现已认识到胚胎干细胞和诱导多能干细胞的致瘤性问题，即胚胎性干细胞植入体内会形成一种混合性胚胎肿瘤：畸胎瘤。所以人们设想通过诱导分化的方法将胚胎性干细胞分化成特定的组织细胞再用于相应的治疗，以避免胚胎性干细胞治疗的致瘤风险。于是，人们将着眼点放在如何纯化分化的细胞，即如何将未分化的胚胎性干细胞从治疗用的分化细胞中去除。同时，人们推测 iPS 细胞治疗的另外一个风险因素来自于外源性的诱导因子。为此，如何优化 iPS 细胞的诱导因子也成为了一个规避干细胞治疗风险的研究热点。基于此观点，人们做了许多工作，包括临床试验。比如日本对视网膜变性病人实施了首例干细胞治疗。但是，紧随其后的第二例视网膜变性病人的预定治疗却被停止，原因是发现了预期用于治疗的细胞存在风险性的基因突变。此临床例证说明人们在对于引起干细胞治疗的基因突变问题尚缺乏了解的情况下，只能是通过盲人摸象式的试探与猜测来评估干细胞治疗的风险与灾难，不能够科学地规避风险，因此难以掌控如何获得安全的治疗细胞。只有将临床尝试建立在成熟阐明干细胞治疗中基因突变机制的基础理论之上，其临床安全性才能够得到合理的保障。

人们对干细胞治疗的初心是要得到足够数量行使正常生理功能的细胞，用其修复、重建或替代病变的组织器官。因此，获得足够数量用于治疗的正常细胞是干细胞治疗的前提。并且，各种组织器官的各种特定功能是以其相应的细胞分化为基础的。没有分化细胞就没有组织器官的生理功能。所以干细胞治疗的重点还是细胞的分化。既然胚胎干细胞和诱导多能干细胞具有的致瘤性(畸胎瘤)问题使其不能直接用于机体植入,那么定向性干细胞和分化细胞是否植入人体就安全了呢？要回答这一问题还是得回到干细胞治疗的处理过程。胚胎干细胞是在胚胎早期阶段的特定时间、特定位置与空间形成的时限短暂的未分化细胞,在正常成体中并不存在这种细胞形式。而 iPS 细胞则是人为地通过外源性因素诱导已经分化的体细胞形成的一种在正常体内并不存在的多能性干细胞。因为胚胎性干细胞对环境信号程序与分化进程时间程序有着严格的要求,任何程序的紊乱都会带来异常的严重后果,人为造成的畸胎瘤就是胚胎性干细胞在错误的时间与错误的地点和空间体内植入的结果。所以要想通过胚胎性干细胞得到足够数量的治疗用分化细胞,目前的途径是进行体外的扩增。然而多细胞高级生物机体为了维护其自身的稳定建立起了严苛的细胞自稳机制。而这种细胞自稳机制的全套完整功能体系存在于每个正常的细胞自身,并且自然规律赋予了每个正常细胞通过这种细胞自稳机制在细胞处于非生理性圆缩的状况下须步入圆缩凋亡的命途,以维护机体整体的安全性。所以,无论在体内还是在体外,多细胞生物分化的体细胞都恪守固有的细胞自稳特性,也就是胚胎性干细胞一旦进入分化,无论是定向性干细胞还是分化细胞都严格地受到细胞自稳机制的管控。细胞的铺展、生长因子以及生长因子的可及性限控机制构成了可增殖体细胞的增殖调控中心环节。机体为了避免细胞在圆缩情况下逃脱这 3 个基本增殖调控环节的制约,又形成了其固有的、以圆缩凋亡和致死性 MIGI 为细胞分子生物学基础的细胞自稳机制,从而限制细胞的恶性增殖与异位种植。正常细胞一旦由于非生理性因素造成圆缩发生(图 2-1),即使能够通过再铺展逃过了圆缩凋亡,但构成 MIGI 重要分子基础的单链 DNA 失去其结合蛋白(RPA、POT1)保护的事件,也将使其无法躲过接下来的灾难性命运——MIGI(图 2-1)。更为重要的是,无论对于胚胎干细胞、诱导多能干细胞、间充质干细胞还是脐血干细胞,只要细胞在获取、诱导去分化与诱导再分化、培养与扩增等任何过程中存在体外处理的环节,就避免不了圆缩事件的发生。因而这些分化细胞若用于治疗,也就逃脱不了圆缩凋亡和 MIGI 的命运。后者包括衰老、致瘤,以及大规模基因突变形成的致病风险。目前,因缺乏对每一个治疗用分化细胞的无损伤性安全风险检测方法,只能靠细胞群体的基因变异和突变细胞潜伏风险以及治疗后的有限观察时间内的致病暴露性来推断细胞治疗的安全性。但是,致病的短暂未暴露性,并不能排除远期的安全风险。所以,基因变异的后续演化致病性"潜伏期"长短,无疑是构成治疗安全性的高风险因素。这种 MIGI 带来的风险也就自然形成了干细胞治疗的安全性瓶颈。如何突破这一安全性瓶颈,是对干细胞治疗的一项巨大挑战(图 2-1)。

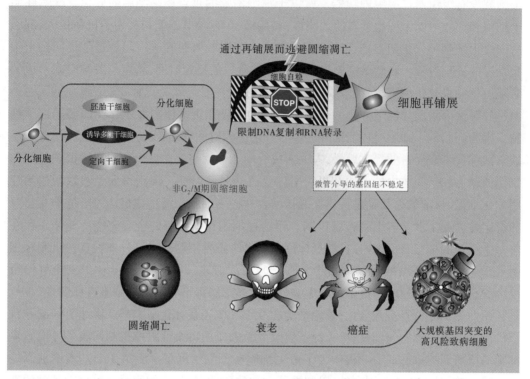

图2-1　实体干细胞体外分化处理的命运

二　癌细胞的特征是基因组稳定还是基因组不稳定

　　基因组不稳定性导致的基因突变是癌症产生的重要原因（由化学、生物致基因突变性致癌因素、紫外线和放射线辐照直接引起的除外）。这已经成为癌症领域几十年长期研究得出的共识。然而，已癌变细胞基因组的稳定性状态究竟是如何呢？换句话说，癌细胞的基因组是稳定的还是不稳定的？一直是存在争议的重要谜题。如何从机制上阐明这一问题，对于认识癌症的发生发展，以及制定正确的临床治疗策略与方案都是至关重要的。MIGI的实验和其原理提示，在细胞癌变阶段，基于MIGI原理的基因组不稳定性是致癌的关键因素。而癌细胞一旦形成，其生长方式、基于MIGI的基因组状态以及癌细胞的代谢方式三者就形成了必然性的耦联，即出现了两种类型的生长、代谢与基因组稳定性模式。一种类型是癌细胞通过有氧酵解模式，使癌细胞基因组变得稳定，也就是避开了圆缩凋亡和MIGI，此时的癌细胞能够以快速、杂乱无序、摆脱机体生理性细胞自稳调控机制的恶性生物学行为生长；而另外一种类型是癌细胞以接近于正常代谢并受控于圆缩凋亡构成的细胞自稳机制的模式生长增殖，细胞一旦发生圆缩，其基因组即会失去

DNA 单链结合蛋白的保护进入 MIGI 状态。故其只能以近似于良性肿瘤的方式生长，否则，难逃圆缩凋亡、急性致死性 MIGI、衰老性死亡、非急性致死性 MIGI（大规模基因变异）以及表观遗传学改变的命运结局。当然，近似于良性肿瘤生长方式的癌细胞也可通过非急性致死性 MIGI 或表观遗传学途径将其代谢模式转变进化成为前一种类型。

　　无论如何，癌细胞进化的目标是为了新的适应和生存。如果进化的目的是为了灭亡，那还会有持续的进化吗？而基因组若不能适应新的快速增殖的生长模式，致使其频繁发生 MIGI 导致的随机的大规模基因突变，其后果必定是致死性的。反之，只有癌细胞适应新的生长存活方式，并且能维持其基因组的稳定性，则癌细胞才能够在保持其恶性生物学行为（如侵袭、扩散和转移）的情况下，得以持续稳定地繁衍生存。因此，无论何种遗传改变，癌细胞若要能够以恶性生物学行为的方式生长，就必须走有氧酵解的代谢之路，以逃过圆缩凋亡及 MIGI 的致死作用，此时的基因组也就自然是趋于稳定的。HeLa 细胞就是最典型的代表。这株细胞自 1951 年从美国妇女的宫颈癌组织取出建系以来，经历了近 70 年的存活，在遍布全世界难计其数的实验室中进行着培养、繁殖与传代，现已成为了癌症等生物医学研究的重要工具。与其相关的科研成果，已获得了 5 次诺贝尔奖。这个细胞的伟大之处，不仅在于已经对人类的健康事业发挥了重要的作用，而且她的神奇正在并仍将带给我们认识生命与癌症本质的更大启迪。虽然，迄今 HeLa 细胞的繁殖数量已超过 5 000 万吨，相当于 100 多座纽约帝国大厦，然而，其基因组却非常稳定，甚至于 2013 年有研究发现，其在点突变方面都呈现出惊人的基因组稳定性。无疑，这种具有典型恶性生物学行为的癌细胞，也在通过代谢模式的改变逃避 MIGI 和圆缩凋亡而得以稳定存活的机制方面，给了我们至关重要的提示。

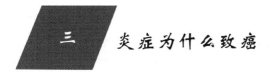

三　炎症为什么致癌

　　并不是每个人的一生中都会接触到致癌剂量的诱变剂和放射线，但是几乎没有哪一个人的一生中没有发生过任何种类的炎症，包括生物性炎症（如呼吸道感染引起的感冒，以及肺、肝、肾、胃、肠、脑、鼻、咽、口腔、四肢、皮肤等各种生物感染性炎症）、物理性炎症（如各种创伤性炎症，可以是开放性与非开放性）、化学性炎症（如各种化学品损伤包括药物性炎症）、混合性炎症（如物理、化学合并生物感染等）。炎症除了其共同特征——红、肿、热、痛之外，还有一个重要特点是由炎症部位组织结构发生变化引起的细胞圆缩与脱落。临床医学实践所依赖的一个非常重要的学科叫脱落细胞学。它可以在细胞水平上与病理学相辅相成，为临床提供最直接的客观诊断依据。可见圆缩与脱落细胞——这种存在于高级多细胞生物的寻常事件，其重要性是不言而喻的。然而，这一事件深层的 MIGI 因素从细胞分子生物学层面为我们认识为什么炎症致癌提供了线索。正因为各种炎症与损伤是造成 MIGI 的重要源头，这对于我们积极地预防和治疗炎症，尤其是防御性地干预反复发作的慢性炎症引起的细胞圆缩与再铺展的往复发生具有重要的临床意义。

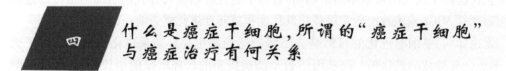

四　什么是癌症干细胞，所谓的"癌症干细胞"与癌症治疗有何关系

现在人们认为"癌症干细胞"是造成癌症转移、复发和放化疗耐受的罪魁祸首。在所谓的"癌症干细胞"的定义中有一个最重要的概念即无限增殖能力。这种能力无疑是铸成癌细胞转移的基础。但是如何用这一概念来解释耐药和复发却是一个不甚明了的问题。除了反复化疗造成的药物诱导性抗药机制建立起的癌细胞获得性或诱导性耐药之外，体内癌细胞总的初始性抗拒放化疗的规律性是：越是处于增殖水平较低的、分化状态较高的细胞，越是对于放化疗表现出较高的耐受性；与之相反，越是处于增殖活跃的、分化状态较低的细胞，越是对于放化疗表现出较高的敏感性（诱导性抗拒除外）。这也是为什么放化疗易于造成骨髓抑制、脱发、黏膜溃疡等机体定向干细胞丰富的快速增殖更新组织损伤的原因。而所谓的"癌症干细胞"除了其类似于机体定向干细胞的高增殖活性之外，更重要的是还具有类似于胚胎干细胞的有氧酵解代谢模式。这就使其更具有了除抗圆缩凋亡和 MIGI 能力之外最棘手的在恶劣生存微环境条件下的"休眠性"以及长期传统治疗后的诱导性抗放化疗能力。再者，虽然由于基因的遗传学变异，使得"癌症干细胞"有别于胚胎干细胞，具有了"顽强去分化"的干性转变，但是由于表观遗传学改变而使其代谢发生转化，具有了干性的癌细胞，又可根据表观遗传学可逆性改变的特点，变回到类似于良性肿瘤的代谢模式，这就为治疗结果的判定以及治疗方案的确立须依据病情的变化而进行动态调整的要求提供了理论依据与指导原则。所以说"癌症干细胞"实际上是一个模糊的概念，广义地讲，一切能够形成致死性转移癌的细胞都应当属于所谓的"癌症干细胞"的范畴。如果抛开致死性转移，那所谓的"癌症干细胞"也就失去了意义。所谓的"干"，其主要内涵为"起源于"。一个致死性转移癌可以直接起源于具有高度恶性生物学行为（快速增殖、浸润性生长、远处转移等）的癌细胞，也可将来自于虽然癌变过程已经完成（癌变所需的最小数量癌基因或抑癌基因的突变），但尚未逃脱细胞自稳性机制（MIGI 与圆缩凋亡）限控的癌细胞。后者暂时虽不具有前者的恶性生物学行为，但经过 MIGI 与其他致基因突变与表观遗传学改变的因素作用，随时具有突变成前者的可能性。所以说，前者的干性不容置疑，而后者只要通过代谢的改变越过圆缩凋亡与 MIGI 的凋亡与衰老命路，步入抗细胞自稳的永生化的恶性歧途，就自然获得了致死的干性。也就是说，所谓的"癌症干细胞"可以随时地由所谓的"不具干性"的癌细胞转化而来。而后者更具有放化疗和免疫治疗的抗性。所以，研究设计应对后者干性发展、进化相关事件与后果的防治策略，是治疗癌症或实现"带瘤"生存的关键。这就是本研究形成的概念之所以能够成功地用于指导临床实践的重要原因。

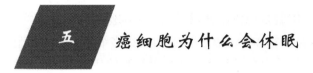

癌细胞为什么会休眠

　　复发是癌症成为难治性顽疾的重要原因。前面讨论了所谓的"癌症干细胞"对于癌症复发的问题。其实,探讨所谓的"癌症干细胞"就不得不涉及另外一个重要概念——休眠。当癌细胞因为某种环境因素的改变,进入到一种既不增殖又不死亡的"睡眠"或静息状态时,就形成了所谓的休眠。癌细胞为什么能够休眠呢？由于治疗、炎症、肿瘤生长等因素造成的微环境破坏与重塑,均可导致癌细胞与其周围的临近细胞和细胞外基质(extracellular matrix,ECM)的关系发生改变。重塑的细胞外基质可以将癌细胞包被其中。前面的段落已经讨论过,细胞外基质对于细胞增殖所依赖的生长因子具有透过性限控作用。此时的癌细胞所处的生存环境如果满足以下条件,即可进入休眠状态。①细胞外基质形成的结构达到了允许小分子营养物质透过而对蛋白质类生长因子进行限制的状态。②癌细胞数量较少,这样可以使得营养物质消耗较少,保证营养物质的消耗量与渗入速率相匹配;细胞外排的有害物质较少,易于耗散(如乳酸),不至于对微环境产生严重破坏性影响。③癌细胞增殖必须依赖常规来源的生长因子(没有生长因子自分泌)。④没有异常(包括基因变异)的生长因子信号通路激活。⑤产能代谢以有氧酵解为主。一旦上述条件造成的癌细胞休眠环境与状态被诸如各种(生物、物理、化学的)炎症与损伤所破坏,癌细胞就会像休眠过后饥不择食的猛兽,疯狂地掠食扩张,从而形成致死性的癌症复发与转移。虽然这种休眠癌细胞由于长期治疗的诱导性作用以及放化疗剂量的极限性,会存在对其放化疗产生抗拒性,甚至对于细胞免疫治疗也是无法可及的,然而,从理论上讲,前面介绍的治疗方案恰恰可以针对这种休眠癌细胞发挥治疗作用,置这些潜伏的癌细胞于死地。

高级多细胞生物怎样构筑起天然的防御机制, 其在癌症预防和治疗方面有何临床意义

　　高级多细胞生物要想存活就需要构筑起机体的天然性防御机制,以维护自身存活的安全性。那么,高级多细胞生物的存活要面对哪些方面的危险呢？最基本的就是两个方面,即外源性的致病因素入侵和内源性的细胞异常生长。为了清除外源入侵的病原体以及由此造成的组织损伤性次级病原物质,机体就演化出了防御性的免疫机制(图2-2);而为了维护正常的组织结构、避免和阻止组织损伤造成的圆缩与脱落细胞的异常生长,机体又演化出了高级多细胞生物所特有的细胞自稳定机制(图2-2)。也就是说,以线粒体、微管、"Junk" DNA(非编码DNA)和细胞核为基础固件要素形成的核压缩方式的细胞

生命调控自稳机制是高级多细胞生物的细胞所独有的。相较于低等单细胞生物,机体细胞以圆缩凋亡和致死性 MIGI 奠定的细胞自稳机制铸成了高级多细胞生物的立命之本。之所以细胞自稳机制会成为高级多细胞生物的立命之本,是由高级多细胞生物的细胞脱落代谢特点决定的,即高级多细胞生物的生命过程无不依赖于细胞的代谢更新(从增殖分化到衰老脱落)。而这种细胞代谢必须是以维持严格的生理性组织结构为前提的,因为只有维持严格的生理性组织结构,各种组织器官才能够行使其正常的生理功能。然而,在自然状态下,高级多细胞生物组织器官的细胞无时无刻不会受到非生理性致病因素的侵袭,因此必然会造成细胞的病理性圆缩与脱落。为了避免圆缩脱落细胞的非生理性种植生长造成的组织生理性结构的破坏,机体进化出了由圆缩凋亡、致死性 MIGI 与黏附选择(如 Integrin 和其他黏附分子家族的组织特异性选择)构成的细胞自稳机制。正是有了这一细胞自稳机制,高级多细胞生物机体才能够阻止脱落细胞(包括正常细胞、良性肿瘤细胞以及类似于良性肿瘤的恶性肿瘤细胞)的疯狂生长,从而避免由此导致的组织器官生理功能丧失的灭顶之灾。否则,非生理性脱落的正常细胞就会像具有侵袭转移性的癌细胞一样,以恶性生物学行为方式全身性地肆意生长,使机体变成一群混沌的无生理功能的失控细胞团。高级多细胞生物如果丧失了高度有机化的器官与生理功能系统,其自身也就不可能存活了。

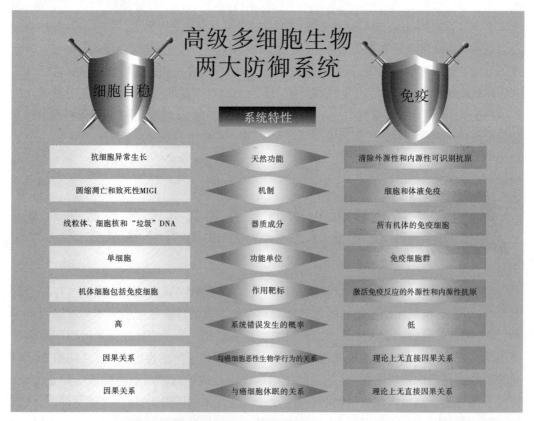

图 2-2　高级多细胞生物两大天然防御系统的主要特性

既然是全身细胞都要受到细胞自稳机制的限控,那么,作为机体组成部分的、决定免疫系统功能的免疫细胞也自然要处于细胞自稳机制的限控之中。如同实体组织细胞,若其遗传系统发生代谢异常(变为有氧酵解代谢为主),将逃脱细胞自稳机制的限控从而生成具有恶性生物学行为的实体肿瘤一样,免疫细胞若通过代谢调控的异常,逃脱了细胞自稳机制的限控则会同样发展成为血液肿瘤白血病(血癌)。除了免疫细胞自身的癌变之外,免疫机制在抵御外部入侵造成的组织损伤方面也与实体肿瘤的发生有着重要的关系。外部致炎性病原因素入侵机体在导致炎症反应性组织损伤的同时,还会造成之前一项不为人们所重视的事件,即体细胞的圆缩。虽然正常代谢的脱落细胞难以逃脱圆缩凋亡的命运,但是,相较于完全脱落的正常代谢细胞,尚处于原位、面临圆缩凋亡的圆缩细胞则较易于获得虽能免于一死却会带给机体潜伏性灾难的重生机会。因为,只要圆缩细胞在圆缩凋亡开启之前的期间内能够得以再铺展,就会逃脱圆缩凋亡和致死性 MIGI 的作用,并且在非致死性 MIGI 的作用下发生大规模的基因与染色体变异,为癌变与衰老奠定基础。因此,即使有细胞自稳和免疫两大天然防御机制来维护机体的安全,各种致病因素造成的组织炎性损伤仍然是终生难以避免的重要致癌事件。只有通过预防病原体的入侵,以及避免和消除各种致炎因素的作用,才可以减少与降低炎性组织损伤事件的发生;并且通过积极、及时、快速、有效的治疗,则可以阻止、减少与降低慢性炎症的发生及其迁延不愈的反复发作。这些预防与治疗措施具有从源头上减少与降低癌变所需基因突变发生概率的重要临床意义。更为重要的是,根据本书所阐明的癌细胞通过代谢模式的遗传学改变演化出逃脱圆缩凋亡与致死性 MIGI 的细胞与分子生物学机制,一种全新的治疗策略与方案在这一理论概念的指导下已成功地得到了临床实践的检验。实现了首个预防和阻止癌细胞恶性生物学行为——侵袭和转移的革命性治疗突破。并且其具有高特异性、低毒副作用、药物费用低廉、给药途径方便的治疗特点。该方法为在维持高生活质量的前提下,延长癌症病人的生命奠定了细胞与分子生物学理论与临床实践基础。

七　体细胞克隆安全吗

许多年前,人们开始进行体细胞的动物克隆,目的是去做一些人们理想的事情。然而,之前对体细胞克隆的安全性缺乏理论上的阐明。本研究提示,在现有方法与技术的操作下,正常体细胞的一次体外传代培养即可由于 MIGI 的原因造成大规模的基因突变,这或许是体细胞克隆难以成功的原因之一。再者,即使这种克隆逃过了致死性基因突变的作用,其随机发生的、MIGI 导致的大规模基因突变也不可能使得克隆后代具有同样的基因与表型,并且其大规模基因突变如同一颗启动的定时炸弹为将来的后续疾病发生埋下了灾难性的遗传学隐患。21 年前诞生的体细胞克隆羊多莉(Dolly)的年轻多病与迫不得已的安乐死,或许令人们至今记忆犹新,并已带给了人们一些有益的和至关重要的启示。

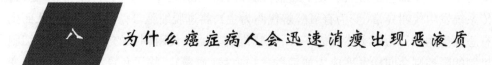

八　为什么癌症病人会迅速消瘦出现恶液质

所谓"恶液质"是指癌症病人极度消瘦以及全身生理功能紊乱和衰竭的一种病理状态。究其原因,癌组织的恶性消耗可谓首当其冲。在恶性生长的癌细胞中,其糖酵解的速率比其正常来源组织细胞的糖酵解速率高出 200 多倍。然而,癌细胞如此高的糖酵解速率与其生长增殖的速率并不匹配,如许多消化系统正常上皮的增殖速度远远大于癌细胞的增殖速度。为什么? 答案在于,癌细胞之所以演化出这么高速率的糖酵解,首先是为了满足其抗细胞自稳机制的恶性存活需要。只有基于这种抗细胞自稳机制的前提,癌细胞才能够得以恶性生长增殖。再者,与这种糖酵解消耗大量葡萄糖形成级联关系的乳酸产生,则构成了癌细胞恶性消耗的另一重要因素。相较于正常细胞,具有恶性生物学行为的癌细胞的乳酸产量远高于正常细胞两个数量级(2 orders)。机体为了避免如此大量乳酸产生导致的堆积性酸中毒,以及补偿大量糖酵解的葡萄糖消耗不得不通过乳酸循环(Lactic acid cycle)(也被称为 Cori 循环,以其发现者 1947 年诺贝尔生理学或医学奖得主 Carl Ferdinand Cori 夫妇的名字命名)进行能量循环代谢。然而,这一过程也是以耗费相应的 ATP 为前提的。因此,在癌细胞高速率的糖酵解、高增加荷载的 Cori 循环以及癌细胞高恶性程度的生长这 3 个方面高能耗的作用下,机体出现恶液质也就在所难免了。当然,由这些高能耗代谢而引发的各种继发性生理生化代谢功能紊乱,自然会起到推波助澜的作用。由此,相较于几十千克重的良性肿瘤,小小的恶性肿瘤竟会引起病人如此严重的恶液质,其原因也就不难理解了。理论上讲,对于一个荷有 0.5 kg 具有高度恶性生物学行为肿瘤的病人,每日所需的进食量至少要达到正常人进食量的 3～4 倍(5 kg 左右)才可以仅仅平衡维持其肿瘤恶性存活的能量消耗,否则,肿瘤将会以消耗机体组织来获取其赖以存活的能量。所以,千万不要试图以限制饮食摄入来饿死癌细胞,因为这样做,饿死的不是癌细胞而只能是病人。这也提示,解决了异质性肿瘤中高度恶性的癌细胞问题,也就为治疗癌症赢得了宝贵的所需时间和机会。

九　为什么异质性是癌症难治的一个重要原因

通过分子遗传学以及 MIGI 的原理来分析癌细胞的异质性,就不难理解,各种癌细胞真可谓是千差万别。像蜘蛛网一样的各种分子信号通路构成了条条大路通罗马的复杂"地图",令人眼花缭乱。虽然,当下针对各种信号通路的靶点发掘可谓是日新月异,但却总也跟不上那"地图"上繁星般的变异花样与速度。但是中国有句成语,叫"万变不离其宗",它哲理性地道出了不管癌细胞如何变化,其选择性适应的结局是要符合这样一个最基本的简单道理:能够存活。因此,从癌症的生存方式上讲,其异质性的划分,无非就是氧化磷酸化为主还是有氧酵解为主这么两种简单的形式。并且仅凭这两种情况不但可以囊括癌症关键性的生物学行为,还能够简捷明了地确定癌症的治疗方案,解决大多癌症的治疗问题。因为每个癌细胞的代谢方式不一样,杀死了有氧酵解为主要代谢方式的原始性放化疗敏感的癌细胞,剩余的接近于正常代谢的原始性放化疗耐受的癌细胞和放化疗诱导的获得性抗性的癌细胞就会成为优势群体,继续生长。而不了解这个原理,接下来的治疗就会陷入"难治"的窘境。如果通过应用以这种代谢模式划分异质性的概念来指导确定临床治疗方案,就可以尽可能地采取局部减少瘤荷的治疗措施(如常规或微创手术等),进一步处理残存的肿瘤。因,此时的肿瘤会以接近良性肿瘤的方式生长,在 BAG 方案的预防和治疗癌症转移的措施保障下,铲除式的外科手术将恰好发挥其独到的治疗作用。

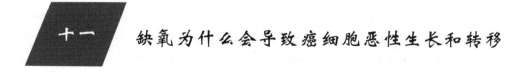

十 为什么癌细胞会走有氧酵解之路

正常细胞在有氧的情况下,会以有氧氧化(氧化磷酸化)的方式进行代谢。细胞走这条三羧酸循环(也被称作 Krebs 循环,以诺贝尔奖得主该循环的发现者 Hans Adolf Krebs 的名字命名)之路能够获得较高的 ATP 产出,即每消耗一分子葡萄糖产生 36 分子 ATP。而许多癌细胞即使在氧气供应充足的情况下,也依然会走一条低产能(一分子葡萄糖生成 2 分子 ATP)的代谢通路,既有氧酵解。这就是著名的以诺贝尔获奖者 Otto Heinrich Warburg 的名字命名的 Warburg 效应。为什么会出现 Warburg 效应?因为,不走三羧酸循环的代谢通路,自然就失去了其关键的 GTP 产生环节。另外,有氧酵解模式的低 ATP 产率也会相应地减少 ATP 向 GTP 的转化。GTP 作为大需求量的构建细胞骨架不可或缺的关键性"建筑"原材料,其大比例的减少对于微管的组装将产生重要的影响。并且 ATP 的减少也会相应地影响到细胞发生圆缩时微管产生压缩力所需的能耗。随着微管组装量的减少,及其产生的核压缩力的减少,癌细胞就可以通过抗细胞自稳,避免圆缩凋亡和 MIGI 带来的致死性和衰老性命运。

十一 缺氧为什么会导致癌细胞恶性生长和转移

原理类似于 Warburg 效应。只不过这种作用是由环境所为,是无氧酵解,而不是有氧酵解。无论是有氧酵解还是无氧酵解，其本质都是糖酵解。缺氧会改变癌细胞的代谢方式，从有氧氧化向无氧酵解模式转变。这种代谢的改变使得原来没有走有氧酵解路径的癌细胞也能够突破原来的生长模式，由近似于良性肿瘤的生长模式转向更具恶性生物学行为的模式生长。一旦缺氧造成的无氧酵解使 GTP 的产出量降低到可逃脱细胞自稳机制的阈值，这种环境驱动的恶性表型就会表现出像有氧酵解一样的效应，即无序生长、侵袭和转移。

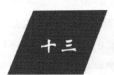

为什么有些肿瘤在其早期即发生远处转移

临床上，许多癌症病人初诊时发现的肿瘤已经是转移性病灶。并且通过现有的技术手段无法检测到原发部位的病变。为什么会出现这种现象？根据机体对脱落细胞的细胞自稳性限控（细胞核压缩导致的转录阻滞性死亡——圆缩凋亡和 MIGI 产生的致死性突变）原理，只要癌细胞其基因突变或表观遗传学改变的结果可以导致代谢的改变，从氧化磷酸化为主转变到有氧酵解为主，就可以逃脱这一细胞自稳性"刹车"机制的作用，此时的癌细胞一旦脱落进入循环系统就可能形成转移性癌灶（当然，黏附与锚定条件可能会起到一定的辅助作用）。所以在癌变形成的早期，只要个别细胞的突变满足了产生这种代谢模式的改变，即可通过逃避圆缩凋亡和致死性 MIGI 的制约能够在循环系统中得以存活，从而发生远处转移。并且其转移灶会呈现出快速生长的恶性表型。此时，原发部位的癌细胞有可能因各种原因造成的存活不适应性选择而消亡；也有可能以低度恶性的表型缓慢生长（原发灶肿瘤与转移灶肿瘤会存在不同的遗传学变异）；还可能随着进一步的基因突变与表观遗传学改变，而表现出滞后性的恶性生长。

为什么一次事件就会造成大规模基因突变的"染色体碎裂"

2011 年 Philip J. 等科学家在 *Cell* 杂志上发表文章报道，通过对慢性淋巴白血病的 DNA 测序，发现了一种由于一次事件而导致大规模基因突变与染色体重排的现象，并将其命名为"染色体碎裂"（chromothripsis）。chromothripsis 一词源自于希腊语，其中 chromo 和 thripsis 分别指"染色体"和"裂成碎片"，整个词义被译成为中文"染色体碎裂"，形容一次事件导致 DNA 的大规模变异的程度。这一现象不断地在后续研究的许多种类的癌症中被证实。虽然此前对这一现象背后的机制不得而知，但观察到这一现象本身即是一次革命性的发现。长期以来，人们一直认为细胞的癌变是由于长时间基因突变逐步累积的结果,而染色体碎裂的发现从观念上颠覆了人们对于癌变的传统认识。2013 年 Aguilera A. 等人在 *Annual Review of Genetics* 发表综述认为"理解染色体碎裂的分子基础将一定会增强我们对基因组不稳定性和其后果的认识""只是现在为时太早,以至于我们还不能够知道其产生的原因"。随着近来研究的广泛展开,出现了几种力求解释"染色体碎裂"机制的模型,包括核小体模型、有丝分裂期间的电离辐射、流产的凋亡以及端粒功能异常等。然而,从细胞圆缩这一多细胞生物最具普遍性与必然性的生物事件所导致的基因组不稳定性,以及细胞的一次圆缩即可从基因和染色体水平上造成大规模灾难性变异的原理和证实性实验上讲,MIGI 无疑对我们认识、解释和阐明染色体碎裂发生的机理提供了详实的线索。

 为什么青少年骨肉瘤病人往往具有外伤史

青少年骨肉瘤是一种恶性程度和致死率极高的骨癌。长期以来的临床资料显示,青少年骨肉瘤的患者往往伴有外伤史。由于对物理性外伤与基因变异性骨癌之间的因果关系缺乏了解,外伤是否是骨癌的一个诱发因素,成为了长期以来争论的焦点问题。随着研究的进展,新的数据为阐明外伤与青少年骨癌发病的关系提供了研究的基础。从基因方面分析,约 33% 的骨癌存在染色体碎裂,这与临床资料报道的约 1/3(33%)的青少年骨肉瘤患者具有外伤史的数据十分吻合,两者之间是否存在因果的联系呢? MIGI 则能够提供解释其关系的线索。外伤的最主要特征就是物理性因素导致的炎症反应。无论何种因素引发的炎症均会造成局部组织结构的破坏,组织微环境的破坏会影响细胞与细胞、细胞与邻近组织的连接,造成细胞的圆缩与再铺展。青少年时期正处在骨骼生长发育阶段,与骨骼生长相关的细胞恰好处于活跃的增殖状态,此时增殖细胞的圆缩与再铺展自然会导致 MIGI 的发生。MIGI 又恰是染色体碎裂形成的基础。所以从理论上讲,外伤与青少年骨癌存在着密切的联系。骨癌是青少年高发的恶性肿瘤,严重威胁着青少年的生命健康。认识青少年骨癌的发病机制对于预防和治疗这种疾病具有重要的临床意义。

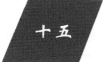 **海弗里克极限是由端粒缩短造成的吗**

1961 年美国解剖学家莱昂纳德·海弗里克(Leonard Hayflick)发现人的正常成纤维细胞在体外培养时,经过 40~60 次群体倍增(population doubling,PD),细胞就会停止分裂。后来,这一现象被称之为海弗里克极限(Hayflick limit),并成为了著名的解释正常细

胞寿命极限的经典假说。然而,当时人们对这种现象的机制并不了解,直到2009年,因获得诺贝尔生理学或医学奖的成果:发现了端粒和端粒酶保护染色体的机制,人们即开始用其解释产生海弗里克极限现象背后的支持机制。即正常体细胞每经过一次染色体复制和有丝分裂,端粒的长度就会有一定量的缩短,当端粒缩短到了一定的长度(尚未有准确数值的报道),细胞就会停止分裂,所以端粒的长度也被称之为"生命的时钟"。但是,科学家也发现了一个问题,老鼠的正常成纤维细胞在经历了20~30次PD之后,仍保留着较长的端粒和高活性的端粒酶(具有维持端粒长度作用的酶),却也会像人的正常成纤维细胞一样停止有丝分裂,并衰老死亡。为什么?人们无法对其做出解释。因发现端粒保护机制而获得2009年诺贝尔生理学或医学奖的得主之一,美国哈佛医学院的杰克·绍斯塔克(Jack Szostak)(另外两位得主分别是加利福尼亚旧金山大学的伊丽莎白·布莱克本,Elizabeth Blackburn,和巴尔的摩约翰·霍普金医学院的卡罗尔·格雷德,Carol Greider)称其为一个好的谜题。因此也有科学家无奈地将这种情况解释为:老鼠的细胞可能跟人的细胞不一样。果真如此吗?大家如果做过细胞培养就不难发现这样一个看似非常普通,而且不得不作为常规操作进行细胞处理的步骤——传代。通常的贴壁培养细胞传代处理的过程是,当培养的正常细胞在培养器皿中贴壁铺展长满之后,要通过某种手段(如最普通也是最经典的处理方式——用胰蛋白酶消化或机械刮落)将细胞从培养器皿壁上剥离下来,形成分散的单细胞悬液或小团片,再根据不同的实验目的进行贴壁种植。于是问题就来了,一旦细胞被剥离脱落,其应力状态立刻发生改变,细胞会因为原来肌动蛋白锚定于细胞外基质和(或)通过细胞间连接建立起来的牵拉张力的骤减以及流体力学的作用而发生圆缩,并且在微管产生的压缩力的作用下,细胞核被剧烈地压缩。此时的细胞面临两种命运。一是如果细胞不能够及时地被再种植贴壁,由于细胞核的压缩、RNA转录的被限制、蛋白质的无从翻译、现存RNA的降解、酶的失活、生化反应的紊乱等级联性灾难事件,将造成悬浮细胞的死亡,即圆缩凋亡(circompactosis)。第二种命运是,即使细胞被及时地再种植贴壁,但是由于细胞核压缩所造成的RPA和POT1等单链DNA结合蛋白与已结合的单链DNA的解离,使得每个处于DNA合成期细胞的80 000~160 000条复制叉处的单链DNA以及端粒处的单链DNA失去保护。后果是单链DNA结合蛋白丧失了其防止错误的DNA二级结构形成以及避免端粒末端融合的重要功能。也就是,在细胞核空间被剧烈压缩的作用下,大量失去保护的单链DNA被暴露于可产生非生理性黏性配对的单链DNA序列并发生相互接触,如此必定急剧增加了链内、链间、染色体内、染色体间碱基错误配对形成DNA错误二级结构和染色体末端融合的机会。由此造成微管介导的基因组不稳定性,并出现相应的大规模基因突变与染色体畸变。的确,我们的实验检测证实,在对经历3次细胞圆缩的人成纤维细胞核型分析时,就检测发现了异常染色体核型的形成(图2-3)。并且,细胞在经历50次左右的圆缩(与Hayflick的群体倍增与passage次数高度吻合),而非50次的群体倍增,培养历时仅约0.8个月(较之Hayflick的5~6个月,缩短了6.25~7.5倍),细胞即停止群体倍增,步入衰老死亡。这些经历2次圆缩/d[即6次圆缩/(PD·3d)]的细胞培养实验结果提示

MIGI 是造成 Hayflick limit 现象的主要原因,而非端粒缩短所致。因其实际倍增次数与得出 Hayflick limit 的倍增次数相差悬殊,与假设完全不符。另外,作者还做了一个非常有趣的实验。将正常人成纤维细胞采用常规条件培养,但唯有其传代方式采用一种作者发明的可避免传代细胞圆缩的"细胞薄膜爬入"技术。按此方法持续培养的细胞于实验 10 个月终止时,细胞虽经历了 100 多次 PD,但亦未出现像常规细胞圆缩性传代培养那样所呈现的衰老死亡现象。这也进一步提示 Hayflick limit 只是体外细胞圆缩所致的一种人为现象与结果,并不能反映细胞的体内生理状况,更不能将其用作解释和说明体内正常细胞衰老与寿命的经典指标。然而,演绎出 Hayflick limit 的细胞培养方法,作为公认的、经典成熟的可重复实验,却恰恰可为 MIGI 的重要作用提供了一个典型的例证。

46条正常染色体核型	88条异常染色体核型	92条异常染色体核型	92条异常染色体核型 (箭头所指为染色体碎片)

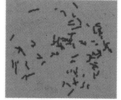 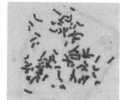 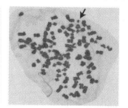

图 2-3　圆缩导致的正常人成纤维细胞核型异常

十六　"垃圾"DNA 的作用是什么,"垃圾"DNA 真的是垃圾吗

　　2005 年 *Science* 杂志创刊 125 周年时,发布了"基因组中的'垃圾'DNA('junk'DNA)有何作用?"的重大科学问题。长期以来,学术界对"垃圾"DNA 究竟是不是垃圾,存在着巨大的争议。因为,随着研究的深入,人们虽然发现可能有些"垃圾"DNA 会参与个别基因的调节,但是仍有很大部分"垃圾"DNA,尤其是"垃圾"DNA 中大量的简单重复序列,无法被证实其功能,所以仍然被认为是"垃圾"。然而,本书作者通过研究发现并提出,所谓的"垃圾"DNA 绝非是"垃圾",其在机体细胞自稳方面有着独特的不可或缺性。也就是说没有"垃圾"DNA,机体的细胞自稳就不可能实现。为什么?由于细胞脱落是高级多细胞生物的自然属性。所以,机体为了防止细胞的原位无序与异位种植性生长,从而实现细胞的自稳,就演化出了 3 个关键性因素:一个是可以产生能够使细胞核被压缩的压力;另一个是细胞在满足生理活动与病理圆缩时细胞核可被压缩的变化空间;第三个是所谓的"垃圾"DNA。细胞在病理性圆缩时,只有通过微管产生的压缩力将细胞核的空间剧烈压缩,使得基因组 DNA 因受压而失去 RNA 转录与 DNA 复制所需的细胞核空间,才能够实现圆缩凋亡与致死性 MIGI 铸成的"刹车"式的细胞自稳。在这一细胞自稳的实施

过程中,"垃圾"DNA 起到了至关重要的"刹车片"作用。因为细胞核膜与 DNA 双螺旋均是具有刚性的固形结构,在细胞发生圆缩时,细胞核会在刚性微管"滑动"方式产生的压力的作用下,以折压性形变的方式被压缩,而并非是细胞核本身的弹性收缩。所以细胞核生理状况下的大小对被折压性形变压缩所需力的大小起着决定性的作用。假如基因组去除掉98.5%的"垃圾"DNA,则细胞圆缩时应当对应于两种理论假设模型:①细胞核按现实的大小被压缩,此时,只有原基因组 1.5% 的 DNA 密度不能够导致形成使 RNA 转录与 DNA 复制受限的核压缩空间,也就不能够实现圆缩凋亡与致死性 MIGI;②若未被压缩的初始细胞核大小为正常细胞核的 1.5%,则细胞核不可能完成按现实细胞圆缩时压缩比率的压缩,因为在此种情况下,仅从细胞核膜、核骨架等细胞核固形成分的空间刚性占位以及压缩过程末端单位面积与体积的微管可产生力的大小与细胞核可受力发生形变的物理条件层面即使得其压缩不可能实现。另外,基因组 DNA 减少为原来的 1.5% 不仅意味着 DNA 密度的大幅降低而且其 DNA 链的缠绕性也随之大幅减少。所以理论上讲,在这种情况下,要达到 RNA 转录与 DNA 复制的"刹车"效应,其细胞核的压缩要远大于真实的压缩比率。再者,在基因组 DNA 减少为实际 DNA 的 1.5% 的情况下,理论上讲,高级多细胞生物为了能够使其细胞分化和组织器官形成而演化出的染色体形成方式、纺锤体形成方式、有丝分裂方式以及遗传方式均不复存在,遗传与生长增殖方式则应类似于原生生物。总之,"垃圾"DNA 在高级多细胞生物细胞的自稳机制的建立与演化中起着基础结构性的、不可或缺的产生空间功能占位效应的关键作用。

十七 化疗为什么会导致癌细胞转移

转移是导致90% 以上癌症病人死亡的重要原因。从传统意义上讲,化疗被认为是预防肿瘤转移的一种治疗手段。然而随着研究的深入,近来人们开始关注化疗造成癌症转移的问题。由于传统化疗缺乏针对癌细胞转移的特异性抑制药物,所以,化疗造成的癌组织微环境破坏会使得癌细胞发生圆缩、MIGI、化疗药物自身导致的基因突变、代谢的有氧酵解转变及其终极的抗圆缩凋亡系列级联事件。并且,非致死剂量的干预微管组装的抗癌药物(如长春碱和紫杉类)可产生与有氧酵解代谢类似的抗圆缩凋亡作用。这些均在突破机体细胞自稳机制上构成了癌细胞转移的细胞分子生物学前提条件。再者,化疗作用造成的癌组织微环境的破坏会使得癌细胞更易于进入循环系统,这无疑为癌细胞的转移创造了便利条件。另外,癌细胞对化疗产生的获得性或诱导性耐药会造成癌组织抗药优先性的细胞异质性重构,这使得在此基础上发生转移以及形成转移灶的癌细胞具备了更大的抗药性。以上提示,在缺乏对转移性癌细胞特异性抑制干预的情况下,任何引起癌症组织微环境破坏的损伤、组织结构修复的抑制以及各种原因产生的炎症均会造成癌细胞的转移。所以,针对癌细胞转移的特异性治疗是癌症治疗的重中之重。

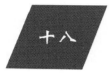

他汀类药物为什么会造成横纹肌溶解症

他汀类药物作为疗效明确的降脂药已在全世界范围内得到了广泛的临床应用。然而,他汀类药物与横纹肌溶解症的关系是各种他汀类药物临床应用的重点注意事项。为什么? 因为横纹肌是构成人体各种运动系统中骨骼肌的组织类型,横纹肌溶解症会造成极其严重的后果。骨骼肌的运动依赖于大量能量的供给。在正常供氧及日常生理活动的情况下,横纹肌主要通过有氧情况下的三羧酸循环(TCA)以氧化磷酸化的形式产出ATP,提供运动所需的能量。其氧化代谢产物主要生成 CO_2 和水。但是,在各种供氧不足因素造成的局部或全身乏氧以及长时间大运动量运动的情况下,横纹肌就会因为氧气缺乏或能量供应不足开启糖酵解的产能代谢通路。虽然糖酵解的产能速度高于有氧氧化,但是其产能效率却远远低于有氧氧化(2 分子 ATP∶36 分子 ATP),只有通过大量糖酵解代谢才能补偿性地提供能量。然而大量糖酵解产能过程却要生成大量的代谢产物乳酸。大量乳酸在骨骼肌细胞内的堆积会造成细胞生化功能的破坏,严重的乳酸堆积会导致灾难性的细胞中毒死亡。由于横纹肌本身不能利用乳酸,所以主要通过乳酸循环(也被称为 Cori 循环,以其发现者 1947 年诺贝尔生理学或医学奖获得者 Carl Ferdinand Cori 夫妇的名字命名)将横纹肌产生的乳酸排入血液经肝再合成葡萄糖循环利用。在横纹肌外排乳酸的环节中,单羧酸转运蛋白 4(monocarboxylate transporter 4,MCT4)起到了关键性的作用,它负责将细胞内的乳酸输送至细胞外。一旦阻滞了 MCT4 的乳酸外输作用将会导致乳酸的胞内堆积,其后果不言而喻。然而他汀类药物恰是 MCT4 的阻滞剂,由此我们就不难理解为什么他汀类药物的副作用会引起横纹肌溶解症了。这提示人们在服用他汀类药物期间应避免各种原因造成的缺氧及过量运动,尤其是对于重病卧床的病人应注意预防发生由于局部压迫和束缚造成的循环障碍性缺血与缺氧。

为什么多细胞生物要有细胞核

高级多细胞生物所固有的特征是组织器官结构的建立,它是维持多细胞高级生物功能的基础。为了能够完成组织器官的新陈代谢以及修复生命过程中不可避免的各种损伤因素对组织造成的损坏,以及维护组织的正常生理结构,机体演化出了由圆缩凋亡和致死性 MIGI 为核心机制构成的防止细胞异常增殖生长的细胞自稳体系。而细胞核、微管、线粒体和"Junk"DNA 则是构成细胞自稳体系的四大核心结构要素。正是由于有了这独特的四大细胞核心结构要素的协同作用,高级多细胞生物才能够形成细胞的自稳机制。有了细胞的自稳机制,正常组织结构才能够得以维持,针对异常免疫原而形成的免疫防御体系也才能够建立。机体才得以保障其繁衍生息。

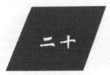

二十 机械力与细胞的增殖以及癌症的发生有什么关系

活跃的细胞增殖加上相应的癌基因与抑癌基因突变就构成了癌症发生的基础。可以说,没有增殖就没有癌症,因为增殖在癌症发生过程中从两方面起到了关键性的作用。一是增殖作用增加了 MIGI 的发生,即增殖的细胞为大规模的基因突变与癌症的进化选择创造了条件,二是只有通过增殖才能够完成致癌相关基因突变的遗传性固定以及癌细胞的形成与生长。而机械性张力的作用恰恰可以通过解除由细胞密度产生的 DNA 活动的细胞核空间限制,并且使得基底膜受张力变化导致的生长因子可及性增强,从而激发细胞的活跃增殖。例如修复损伤的外科皮肤扩张术、外科方式的肢体延长性增高术以及挤压性上皮增生与角质化(俗称老茧)就是基于此细胞分子生物学的作用。在机械张力对机体脏器组织细胞的作用下,各种炎症所造成的细胞圆缩,为 MIGI 带来的致癌性基因突变的进化选择奠定了基础,使癌变更易于发生。所以,采取相应的措施,避免或消除造成脏器超过生理规律的张力性扩张因素(如不合理饮食等因素造成的消化系统异常产气和食物残渣、粪便排泄不畅,以及泌尿系统的液体潴留)。这些措施对于预防癌症的发生具有重要的临床意义。

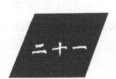

二十一 为什么各种多细胞生物体型大小差异很大而其体细胞大小差异却很小

自然界的生物大到鲸鱼与大象,小到老鼠与跳蚤,虽然个体大小差异悬殊,但其体细胞大小的差别却是微乎其微,为什么? 对于这个问题的回答,之前有各种各样的解释,但是多细胞生物细胞"自稳"的生死攸关性不可不谓之举足轻重。前面谈到,细胞核的大小对细胞的存活至关重要,而细胞的力学结构与受力状态又是决定细胞核大小的重要因素。细胞圆缩产生的压缩力对细胞核的作用是通过压缩 DNA 链在 RNA 转录与 DNA 复制时所必需的功能活动空间、"刹车"式地阻止细胞非正常的致机体于死地的灾难性恶性增殖与生长事件的发生而体现的。机体能否实现这一"细胞自稳"功能,是由细胞的基因组 DNA 分子大小为关键因素的级联作用决定的。细胞依据这一核心因素优化出了其细胞核和细胞体积的适宜大小与比例。违背这一规律的改变都将给机体的生存带来灾难性的结果。因为,假如细胞核变小,基因组 DNA 的生理功能活动空间将无法得到满足;反之,假如细胞核变大,与之匹配的一系列因素都须发生有违自然法则和规律的改变。假设细胞核为球体,如果其轴径增加一倍,则细胞基因组的 DNA 大小需增加至原来的 8 倍才能够与之相匹配。这就意味着"junk" DNA 的分子量、基因拷贝数量、细胞体积、细胞骨架分子等一系列因素都要相应地进行数量增加。然而,这一切都不可能为真,否则,多细胞高级生物体就不可能产生。因为,在此种情况下,机体的循环系统与组织器官的构建、能量供应、细胞受力损伤风险最小化机制、机体运动对组织细胞张力的最小化影响(单位体积内细胞数量对力的分散与分担)、组织更新与损伤修复都将变得不可能。所以,尽管生物个体大小千差万别,但正是由于大自然以线粒体、微管、细胞核与"junk" DNA 四大核心结构要素优化出了多细胞高级生物的细胞与细胞核大小,才使得依赖于细胞自稳系统的各种体型大小的多细胞高级生物得以形成。

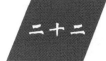

二十二 线粒体为什么要有自己的 DNA 与遗传体系

细胞维持生命活动的过程无不需要能量的供应。线粒体是高级多细胞生物细胞的能源工厂,正常细胞在正常情况下的能量供给主要来自线粒体内的氧化磷酸化反应。由此可见,线粒体对细胞的存活是至关重要的。然而,线粒体作为细胞内的细胞器,不仅自身的复制与更新,而且在其内部进行的产能过程都是在酶的反应催化下完成的。构成酶的主要成分是蛋白质。虽然细胞中的绝大多数参与生化反应的酶蛋白以及组成细胞器的蛋白质是由细胞核的 DNA 编码的,但是线粒体自身的遗传体系基因组直接编码其独特的、与氧化磷酸化供能产出 ATP 密切相关的酶与蛋白产物。总的来讲,酶蛋白属于短寿命的蛋白质,所以要完成其更新,就必须能够及时地从对其编码的 DNA 进行 RNA 的转录。但是当细胞处于细胞周期时相的 M 期,以及由于各种原因引起的正常细胞圆缩时,细胞核中的 DNA 因处于压缩状态,其生理性 RNA 转录活动会受到限制,而此时的细胞却仍然需要供能。在这种情况下,线粒体若没有自己的 DNA 与遗传系统,其后果将不堪设想。

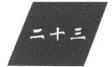

二十三 逆转录病毒怎样通过宿主细胞发生突变

逆转录病毒是一类具有高突变率的 RNA 病毒。这种病毒可以通过病毒自身的逆转录酶,以病毒 RNA 为模板逆转录合成 DNA,然后再将其整合到宿主细胞的基因组中,借助宿主细胞的复制体系来完成病毒的扩增。既然病毒的遗传信息被整合到宿主细胞的基因组,那就意味着影响宿主细胞的 MIGI 效应也同样可能影响到编码病毒遗传的 DNA (图 2-4)。由于各种炎症会引起 MIGI 事件的发生,而且病毒感染本身就是一个致炎因素。所以这将会加大 MIGI 的发生率。不过,病毒的基因组较小,严重的突变将有可能是致死性的无效突变。

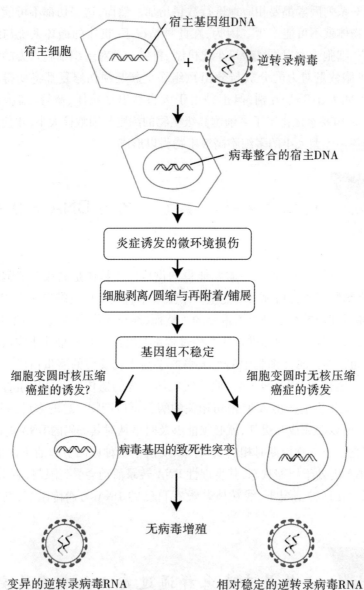

图 2-4 逆转录病毒基因突变理论示意

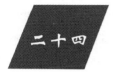

怎样从治疗研究用的混合细胞中去除胚胎性质的干细胞

随着干细胞从最初的发现性研究向目前热切期望的应用性研究转变,人们意识到之前曾寄予厚望的用未分化胚胎性质的干细胞(包括胚胎干细胞以及诱导多能干细胞)植入成体内的疾病治疗方式具有生成恶性肿瘤的巨大安全风险。于是,人们将研究重点转向了把胚胎性质的干细胞诱导分化后再用于体内植入治疗。然而,细胞治疗需要的细胞数量巨大,怎样将已分化的细胞从大量的胚胎性干细胞与分化细胞混合群体中分离纯化,也就是将未分化的胚胎性质的细胞从混合群体中去除却是一项巨大的瓶颈问题式挑战。尽管目前的技术处理手段对于实体干细胞的治疗总体上具有不可避免的安全风险,但是作为研究探索,根据胚胎性干细胞的有氧酵解代谢特点,用类似于本文介绍的药物处理方案就可以提供一条探讨如何本着简便、经济、高效、安全的原则从诱导分化的混杂细胞中去除胚胎性干细胞的环节性解决问题的线索。

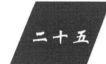

干预糖酵解代谢模式的治疗可能对早孕卵裂球胚胎干细胞的作用与影响

胚胎干细胞是由受精卵生长分裂增殖形成的早期胚胎尚未分化的一种细胞。其代谢特点是以有氧酵解为主。因此,理论上讲,在胚胎发育的胚胎干细胞尚未生长分化为定向干细胞的阶段,对这种有氧酵解代谢模式有干扰作用的药物以及对细胞排酸通道具有抑制作用的药物(包括他汀类与质子泵抑制剂类)均会影响胚胎干细胞的存活与生长。因此,这种干预型治疗是否具有避孕药的终止妊娠药效以及对胚胎发育的危害性作用有待进一步深入研究。

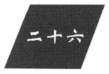

植物原生质体无性育种的机制是什么

植物原生质体无性育种是一种重要的无须外源性转基因的育种手段。跟放射线辐照育种、航天搭载育种等方法相比,植物原生质体无性育种具有经济、安全、易实现、可用于广泛的研究目的等特点,在农作物良种选育、花卉新品种培育等方面得到了广泛的应用。遗憾的是,从原生质体的初次获得到目前为止,虽然经历了半个多世纪的研究,但是对植物原生质体无性育种背后的机制却仍然没有得到阐明。搞清楚其机制,无疑对于植物育种技术的发展具有十分重要的意义。通过对植物原生质体无性育种操作步骤与结果的分析,可以清楚地发现其中的核心规律——细胞圆缩,而细胞一旦圆缩,就不可避免地导致 MIGI 的发生。这正是为什么植物原生质体经分离与培养后会出现遗传性状的变化,且这种改变是不可控的原因。

参考文献

［1］GUO Q,LIAO X L,WANG X W,et al. Cell rounding cause genomic instability by dissocia-tion of single-stranded DNA-binding proteins［DB/OL］. bioRxiv doi:https://doi. org/10. 1101/463653. 2018.

［2］FRISCH S M,FRANCIS H. Disruption of epithelial cell-matrix interactions induces apop-tosis［J］. J Cell Biol,1994,124(4): 619-626.

［3］CHEN C S,MRKSICH M,HUANG S,et al. Geometric control of cell life and death［J］. Science,1997,276(5317): 1425-1428.

［4］GUO Q,TANG W,KOKUDO N,et al. Epidermal growth factor-mediated growth control of confluent mammary epithelial cells cultured on artificial basement membrane［J］. Int J Mol Med,2005,16(3): 395-399.

［5］YAO N Y, O'DONNELL M. SnapShot:The replisome［J］. Cell,2010,141(6):1088-1088.

［6］CREAGER R L,LI Y,MACALPINE D M. SnapShot: Origins of DNA replication［J］. Cell,2015,161(2): 418.

［7］WANG K R,XUE S B,LIU H T. Cell biology［M］. Beijing:Beijing Normal University Press,1990.

［8］MARINO N,NAKAYAMA J,COLLINS J W,et al. Insights into the biology and prevention of tumor metastasis provided by the Nm23 metastasis suppressor gene［J］. Cancer Metasta-sis Rev,2012,31(3-4): 593-603.

［9］SHASHNI B,SHARMA K, SINGH R, et al. Coffee component hydroxyl hydroquinone (HHQ) as a putative ligand for PPAR gamma and implications in breast cancer［J］. BMC Genomics,2013,14 (Suppl 5):1-16.

［10］PINHEIRO C,LONGATTO-FILHO A,AZEVEDO-SILVA J,et al. Role of monocarboxy-late transporters in human cancers: state of the art［J］. Bioenerg. Biomembr,2012,44(1):127-139.

［11］WARBURG O,POSENER K,NEGELEIN E. Über den Stoffwechsel der Carcinomzelle［J］. Biochem Zeitschr,1925,4(12):309-344.

［12］SKLOOT R. The immortal life of henrietta lacks［M］. New York: Crown/Random House, 2010.

［13］AGUILERA A,GARCíA-MUSE T. Causes of genome instability［J］. Annu Rev Genet, 2013,117(1):1-32.

［14］KANSARA M,TENG M W,SMYTH M J,et al. Translational biology of osteosarcoma［J］.

Nat Rev Cancer,2014,14(11):722-735.

[15]YANG J Y,CHENG F W,WONG K C,et al. Initial presentation and management of osteosarcoma,and its impact on disease outcome [J]. Hong Kong Med J 2009,15(6):434-439.

[16]SHAMIR M,BAR-ON Y,PHILLIPS R,et al. SnapShot: Timescales in cell biology [J]. Cell,2016,164(6):1302-1302.

Chapter 1

▶ Therapeutic Principle
and Strategy

1.1　The key survival machinery of advanced multicellular living beings' cells

The nature of life is survival and proliferation, which is suitable to both normal and cancer cells. Cell is the basic unit of constructing living beings. To achieve the goal of survival and proliferation, the cells of advanced multicellular living beings have to complete two fundamental biological activities. Firstly, for survival, a cell needs to establish and maintain a lot of functional systems formed by various proteins, which depend on a core process—RNA transcription. Secondly, for proliferation, a cell needs to double its DNA of bearing genetic codes, which has to undergo four artificially named phases, i. e. , G_1, S, G_2, and M phase. So what is the key limiting factor for RNA transcription and DNA replication? The answer is nuclear size.

As we know, all thingsin nature need space for their existence and activities. This is especially true of the biochemical reactions among various biomolecules that lay the foundation for human cell survival. Although cells belong to the micro-level, the various biochemical reactions in cells are by no means a mixed pot of porridge. DNA is a giant molecule in human cells. The length of DNA molecule in a human cell can reach two meters. Such a long DNA molecule can only be packaged in a nucleus a few microns in size after being highly compacted. Moreover, only when DNA molecules are wrapped and compacted to form chromosomes can duplicated DNA be allocated to two progeny cells during mitosis (M phase). However, DNA in the chromosomal state naturally limits its RNA transcription and DNA replication in space. Therefore, in order to initiate new cell cycle, progeny cells not only need to change DNA from tightly compacted chromosomes to loosely structured chromatin, but also need to unwind the helix and separate double-stranded DNA into single-stranded DNA. All this can only be done when the space of the nucleus becomes large enough. The question is how somatic cells increase their nuclei? The answer is spreading by attachment.

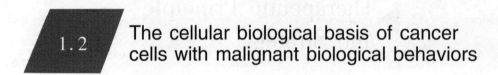

1.2 The cellular biological basis of cancer cells with malignant biological behaviors

When the cell has just finished the M-phase division and become two daughter cells, the cell is round, and does not establish any connection with its surrounding extracellular matrix and other adjacent cells, and the DNA is also compacted. With the attachment and spread of daughter cells and the establishment of connections with other adjacent cells, the nucleus begins to enlarge, DNA changes from chromosome to chromatin, and cells begin to grow, and then the next cell cycle starts. This is the mode of normal cells' growth and proliferation in physiological state. How do cancer cells with malignant biological behaviors grow and proliferate? In other words, why a cancer cell can grow in an invasive and metastatic mode? To answer this question, we have to focus on the nuclear size, which is the key clue to cell growth. As experienced doctors know, an enlarged nucleus is one of the most prominent characteristics of cancer cells, which is the hallmark of diagnostic parameters and suitable for the diagnosis of all kinds of malignant tumors including solid tumors and blood tumors leukemia. Why? As we mentioned earlier, only the enlargement of nucleus can make RNA transcription and DNA replication proceed, cells can survive and proliferate. Moreover, an enlarged nucleus is the key factor not only for a cancer cell's survival and proliferation but also for its invasive growth and distance metastasis. This raises a further question. Is there any difference between the mechanism of nuclear enlargement of normal cells and that of cancer cells with malignant biological behaviors? The answer is yes.

Shape change of all things in the natural world depends on the action of force. The nuclear shape and size of a cell are also determined by force. There are two main kinds of forces in a human cell. One is compacting force generated from microtubules, another, pulling force, from actin filaments. It is just the proper equilibrium of the two forces that maintains the stability of cell growth under the control of physiological orders.

When a normal cell spreads through attachment to extracellular matrix, the pulling force applied by actin filaments counteracts the compacting force by microtubules. Under such circumstances, the two forces achieve a normal equilibrium, which makes the nucleus to be physiologically enlarged so as to fulfill the requirement for RNA transcription and DNA replication. Once the equilibrium of force is lost by breaking the junctions on which the actin filaments depend to generate the pulling force, and compacting force generated by microtubules plus the interfacial tension will become the dominant power of controlling cellular shape and nuclear size. Under this condition, the cell rounding and drastic nuclear compaction will happen (Figure 1-1). In contrast, a cancer cell can maintain the enlarged nucleus (Figure 1-2) during no attachment to the matrix so as to be able to survive in circulation system, and to realize invasion and metastasis. What makes a cancer cell have the characteristic different from a normal cell? As long as we grasp the thread that nuclear size determines not only a cell's life-and-death but also ability to metastasize, the answer will naturally emerge.

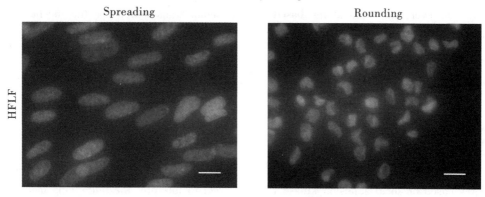

Figure 1-1   The nuclear sizes of human fetal lung fibroblasts

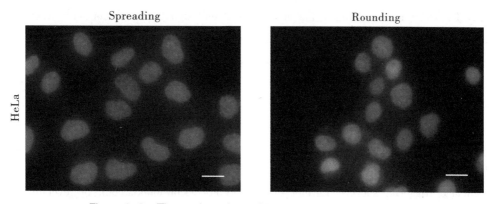

Figure 1-2   The nuclear sizes of human cervical cancer cells

1.3   Circompactosis—the key part of autostabilisis

If a cancer cell has left its primary lesion site and metastasized to a distance organ, it is certain that the cell has successfully survived the autostabilic crisis in a circulation system. This raise a question why a cancer cell can evade the autostabilisis. The answer is the cancer cell acquired the ability to resist circompactosis, which refers to a kind of cell death due to the nuclear compaction of a rounded cell. Here, circompactosis as a new concept has to be introduced to reveal the underlying mechanism of metastasis, because people have formerly observed a phenomenon of cell death, named "anoikis", by which normal cells and some cancer cells without the ability to metastasize will die due to the cellular detachment from their attached extracellular matrix. Although resistance to anoikis was believed to be a prerequisite for cancer metastasis, yet the later researches on uncovering the underlying mechanism of anoikis was almost all focused on the causality between signal transduction and anoikis because of the definition of anoikis. However, the explanations based on the signal transduction for the mechanism of anoikis cannot account for the question why a cell will die just as the cell becomes semi-rounded rather than completely detached. Answering the question is a principle issue which has great significance for investigating the therapeutic strategies to cure cancer. It is just for this reason that the concept of circompactosis was introduced here. And it can exactly elucidate the puzzle in the both sides of pathological phenomenon and mechanism of cell-molecular biology.

Although the viewpoints of cell signal transduction, which is represented by the kernel pathway based on focal adhesion kinase (FAK), tried to interpret the underlying mechanism ofanoikis, yet none of them could account for the key issues about cell survival in the process of anoikis. For example, according to the viewpoints of cell signal transduction, only when a cell was detached from the ECM, the anoikis signaling would be triggered. However, this is not the case. As long as a normal cell becomes semi-rounded, even though it keeps attachment to the ECM, it still cannot escape from the fate of death. Moreover, the conventionally believed mechanism of anoikis cannot interpret the following important issues either. Firstly, since anoikis is believed as an event triggered by signaling of cell detachment, why do a normal cell not undergo apoptosis during a considerable period of time (several hours) after detachment, as long as the cell can get an opportunity for reattachment and re-spreading. In other word, what is the signaling effect of triggering anoikis? Further, even if the process of anoikis could be reversible, what would be the reversible signaling pathway? Secondly, if a cell detachment could trigger the signaling pathway of anoikis, why does a normal cell in a suspension cell sphere not undergo anoikis under the condition of no attachment to ECM? Exactly, what is the effect of cellular attachment to ECM in anoikis? Thirdly, how long can a normal detached cell avoid "anoikis" by re-spreading, and why? To answer these questions, we have to go back to the issues about RNA transcription.

It is well known that the physiological functions of cells cannot be maintained without various biochemical reactions that rely upon various proteins to take part in. This provides a key clue to clearly understand the mechanism underlying "anoikis". When a normal cell undergoes a process of rounding, its nucleus will get into the state of compaction. Under this condition, the RNA transcription will be limited. Thus, there cannot be corresponding proteins to be translated. As a result, the short-lived proteins that play the key roles in modulating metabolic biochemical reactions cannot be well replenished either, which can lead to a fatal catastrophe of severe biochemical disorders unless the cell can obtain an opportunity of re-attachment and re-spreading within a certain period of time. All of these suggest that the conventional explanations based on signaling pathways cannot answer the question why the notion of "anoikis" cannot interpret the phenomena of time-delayed cell death and time-limited cell revival. Therefore, the concept of circompactosis has to be introduced not only to elucidate the causality between the phenomenon and nature of cell-rounding, which is involved in the detached and none-detached cells, but also to indicate the key clue of investigating the mechanism of cancerous metastasis and invasion.

1.4   The relationship between epithelial structure and cancer cell growth

Since more than 90% of human malignant tumors occur from epithelial tissues, the structure of epithelial tissue should certainly take some important roles in maintaining normal cell growth in an orderly way, and in forming the malignant biological behaviors of cancer cells. Therefore, investigating the function of tissue structure may provide important clue to understanding how a cancer cell acquires the ability to grow in the disorderly malignant manner.

A normal epithelial cell has two poles. One is apical pole, and another is basal pole which attaches to the basement membrane to support the cell growth and proliferation. Besides the characteristics of polar structure, a normal epithelial cell also forms some junctions with the adjacent cells, such as tight junction, gap junction, belt junction, bridge junction and semi-bridge junction. Every kind of junction has its corresponding function. The tight junction located in the apical-lateral side plays a sealing role in preventing large molecules to pass through. In the opposite pole, various growth factor receptors are located in the basal and basal-lateral sides. Thus, growth factors can only bind their corresponding receptors by crossing the basement membrane, which plays an important role in limiting the accessibility of growth factors to their receptors. It is in this way that the binding of growth factors to their receptors can realize stimulating normal cell's growth. Also, based on the polar structure, epithelial tissue establishes the machinery for controlling normal epithelial cells' growth. But, as a cell falls into carcinogenesis and further progresses in malignant grade, it will lose its polar structure and presents a tendency of rounding. As a result of the breakage of cellular polarity and basement membrane caused by cancer malignant biological behaviors, the tissue structure is totally out of limiting and controlling the accessibility of growth factors to their receptors. This turns into an important factor to promote the disorderly and out-of-controlled growth of cancer cells. To further understand the effect of issue structure on cell growth-control, we have to clarify a concept of cell "contact inhibition".

The contact inhibition refers to a phenomenon that the normal cells in monolayer culture will stop growth when they reach a confluent state. In contrast, cancer cells are not limited to this nature so that they can grow in an overlapped manner. Why isso? The answer is that the growth and proliferation of normal cells depend on the effect of growth factors. Under normal conditions, growth factors cannot go through tight junctions to bind their receptors located in the basal and basal-lateral sides and therefore they cannot generate the signaling effect of stimulating growth on the cells. The results of the author's previous researches suggested that the so-called contact inhibition, in fact, is merely an artificial phenomenon of cultured cells under certain circumstances in vitro, and it does not exist in vivo. If we make an impermeable bottom of a dish culturing normal cells in contact inhibition be locally permeable to the growth factors, we can see an interesting phenomenon that the cells on the impermeable part remains in contact inhibition while the other cells present a state of actively overlapped growth. For cancer cells, due to the destruction of cell junction structure and loss of polarity, as well as the abnormal activation of growth factor autocrine and/or kinase related to growth signal transduction caused by mutation, the cells can always be in the corresponding state of activation of growth signal pathway, so there is no contact inhibition. In conclusion, genetic and epigenetic variations in various ways can lead to changes in normal tissue structure and cancer cell's rounding. If the cancer cells acquire the ability to evade circompactosis in such case, they will present the malignant phenotype, such as rapid growth, poorer differentiation, evasion, and metastasis. However, malignant tumor cells tending to grow in a benign way (depending on external growth signal stimulation, growth slowly, well differentiated, non−invasive and non−distant metastasis) can hardly escape the fate control of circompactosis. Clinically, the more poorly differentiated cancer cells tend to become rounded, and the more easily they fall out of cancer tissue. This phenomenon corresponds to its notorious malignant biological behaviors, invasive growth and distant metastasis. Originally, cell exfoliation is an unavoidable biological event in multicellular organisms. In order to maintain its own stability, prevent abnormal growth in situ and ectopic planting growth of exfoliated cells, advanced multicellular living beings have evolved a cellular self-limiting and self-stabilization mechanism, circompactosis, caused by nuclear compaction of rounded cells.

So, in addition to the RNA transcriptional blockade and circompactosis caused by nuclear compaction talked above, what other important effects does nuclear compaction have on cells? The answer is yes. As we know, a normal cell attaching to the ECM will becomes rounded only in the M phase of a cell cycle. As long as the daughter cell enters G_1 phase, it will start to grow via attaching to the ECM again. However, the normal cells growing in vivo or cultured in vitro will become rounded under the non-physiological conditions, such as suffering from various inflammation and tumors or being treated by passage, respectively. At S phase, the cells need to separate their double-stranded DNA helixes into unwound single-stranded DNA. In such case, if the normal cells encounter the events of causing cell rounding and drastic unclear compaction, what kind of impact will the events make on the regrowth of the cells? The question will be investigated follows.

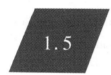

1.5   The catastrophic effect of nuclear compaction on DNA protection mechanism

We can know, from the above, that the nuclear compaction can limit DNA synthesis. However, this is just the tip of the iceberg in terms of the effect of nuclear compaction on DNA activities. It is more surprising that the nuclear compaction can cause the damage of DNA structure and then change the cellular biological behaviors. Because both of DNA and protein are the biological macromolecule compounds, they all have the chemical property of conformational change. This will naturally draw forth the following issues. In Sphase, the prerequisite of DNA replication is that the cell has enough nuclear space so as to avoid mispairing of cohesive base pairs, insure separation of single-stranded DNA chains, and form replication forks. The replication process needs replisome composed of a number of proteins to take part in. Among them, replication protein A (RPA), as a single-stranded DNA binding protein, plays a key role in maintaining the stability of replication forks, and preventing the single-stranded DNA from formation of erroneously secondary structures including the improper ligation in and between chromosomes. However, due to the intense nuclear compaction caused by cell rounding, the conformation of single-stranded DNA and RPA will be changed. Will this affect the combination of the two? If the combination is affected, RPA will lose its protective function, and the consequences will be catastrophic for cells. Whether this hypothesis is true or not, it depends on the following experimental tests to confirm it.

1.6 Significance of establishing the method of "cell in situ Electrophoresis"

In order to test and prove the hypothesis that nuclear compaction can affects the sequence-nonspecific binding of single-stranded DNA and RPA, the experiments have to be performed under the condition of non-broken state of the nuclear compaction. But now all available methods, such as the DNA mobility shift assay, and chromatin immunoprecipitation (ChIP), cannot fulfill the requirement of the test, because these methods need to make the tested cells broken first and then obtain the DNA-protein samples to perform the further complex analyses. In view of the limitations of the above-mentioned methods, the author developed and established a new technical method, Cell in situ Electrophoresis (CISE), to fulfill the requirement of the test. The schematic of CISE is shown as Figure. 1-3. Because human DNA chains belong to macromolecules, they cannot migrate out of the cell with micropore-treatment. As a result of the anchorage effect of the bound DNA, the RPA binding to single-stranded DNA can be still kept in a cell undergoing electrophoresis with some degree of electric-field-force strength. On the contrary, the unbound RPA will migrate out of the cell under the force of electric field. Thereafter, the binding state of RPA can be confirmed by flow cytometric examination for the remained RPA in the cells that have undergone CISE. Based on this technology, the hypothesis was proved, which not only gives the key clue to a series of important biological puzzles but also provides theoretical basis for further guidance of the subsequent clinical practice.

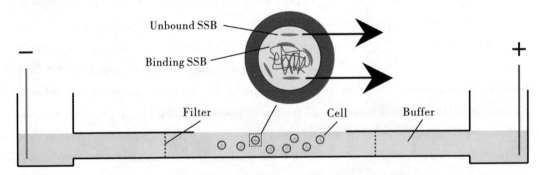

Figure 1-3   The schematic diagram of Cell in situ electrophoresis

1.7   Microtubule–induced genomic instability caused by catastrophic cell rounding

It is well known that there are a large number of complementary DNA repeats in highly compacted nuclei. Because of the dissociation of the binding of RPA to single–stranded DNA, single–stranded DNA loses the important protective role of RPA to prevent the formation of erroneous secondary structures. At the same time, the drastic compaction of nuclear space greatly increases the accessibility of complementary base sequences within and between single–stranded DNA strands. This will inevitably lead to complementary single–stranded DNA mismatches within and between chromosomes, thus forming the wrong secondary structure. Although there are some DNA repair mechanisms in cells, yet, the ability to repair is limited by the degree of error. Otherwise there will be no concept of lethal mutation. Furthermore, there are 40,000 to 80,000 replication origins in every human cell. Without such a large number of DNA replication origins, cells would not be able to complete more than 3 billion base pairs of a large amount of DNA replication in a cell cycle. It also means that during DNA replication, 80,000 to 160,000 single–stranded DNA strands at 40,000 to 80,000 replication forks in a cell is protected by RPA. Once a cell encounters a nuclear–compaction event caused by non–physiological cell rounding, such a large number of single–stranded DNA may lose the protection of RPA. The consequences are doomed to be catastrophic – either leading to cell death (lethal gene mutation) or DNA damage (non–lethal gene mutation, even chromosomal aberration) that cannot be restored, although not immediately lethal.

The occurrence of events and the existence and concepts, which may have the same principles, are the characteristics and laws of nature. Coincidentally, this study further found that telomere protection 1 (POT1) is another capable–of–causing–cell–catastrophe factor similar to RPA binding characteristics. POT1 is also a single–stranded DNA binding protein, which together with other proteins forms a six–protein telomere protein complex (shelterin), which plays a vital role in protection, maintenance and extension of telomeres. Telomere is a protective DNA sequence located at the end of chromosome, which plays a key role in protecting chromosome, maintaining normal structure of chromosome and stability of genome. Similar to RPA, nuclear compaction caused by cell rounding can also lead to the dissociation of POT1 and its binding telomere–single–stranded DNA. One of the key roles of telomere–protective proteins is to prevent the end–to–end fusion of chromosomes and the formation of aneuploidy. Therefore, the loss of telomere and the DNA damage caused by the dissociation of POT1 and RPA from their bound DNA will theoretically produce a cumulative DNA−damage effect of $1+1>2$, which will undoubtedly cause catastrophic DNA damage to the rounded cells. The experimental results have proved it.

Inconclusion, the abnormal cell rounding and nuclear compaction of normal cells will produce microtubule−induced−nuclear−compaction effect, including the limitation of RNA transcription, circompactosis, and MIGI. The effect of MIGI can cause gene mutation, chromosome aberration, and aneuploid formation, which results in immediate cell death or non-immediate cell senescence. Nevertheless, cancer cells can escape the autostabilic effects through whatever forms of gene mutation and/or epigenetic changes, so as to evade nuclear compaction, maintain cell's survival after cell rounding, and make invasion and metastasis possible. Thus, the investigation comes back to the focus of question again — what is the mechanism of maintaining nuclear enlargement after cell rounding?

1.8 The biochemical mechanism of evading autostabilisis

All shape changes in nature are due to force. The nuclear enlargement also belongs to the category of shape change. Talked above, there are two kinds of balancing forces determining nuclear shape and size. One is the pulling force generated by actin, another is the compacting force generated by microtubules. Once the indispensable factors of generating pulling force via actin is changed by damaged cell−cell junctions, broken adhesion of cell−ECM (extracellular matrix), as well as reduced tissue stretch tension, the compacting force will be turned into the dominated force and the nuclear size will be compacted with cell rounding (Figure 1−1).

Since the compacting force comes from microtubules, the changes of microtubules will influence the compacting force. Indeed, when the normal human fibroblasts were treated with vincristine (VCR), a drug as a tool to inhibit assembly of microtubules, the nuclear compaction that should happen under no drug treatment was inhibited (Figure 1−4).

Furthermore, the author designed a cell−suspension−culture experimental device and completed a unique drug experiment. Normal human fibroblasts were divided into drug treatment group and control group. The treatment group was treated with vincristine, a traditional anticancer drug that inhibits microtubule assembly. Flow cytometry was used to detect the circompactosis. Compared with the control group, the circompactotic rate of cells treated with vincristine decreased significantly. So, can cancer cells avoid the nuclear compaction by changing the assembly of microtubules, so as to evade circompactosis? If the answer is yes, what is the underlying mechanism? This also needs to analyze the biochemical elements of microtubule assembly.

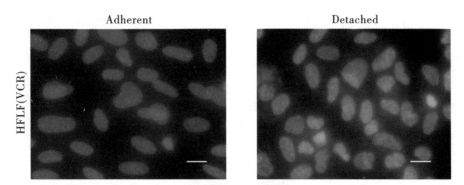

Figure 1-4　The nuclear sizes of HFLFs treated with vincristine (VCR)

Tubulin and guanosine triphosphate (GTP) are the two most important elements for the assembly of microtubules. Without adequate GTP, microtubules can not be assembled properly. If the microtubule assembly that produces compacting force cannot be fulfilled, can the nucleus of cancer cells escape from being compacted when the cells are rounded? If so, how can cancer cells reduce GTP production?

In the biochemical energy metabolism, there is a kernel course of energy production, which is calledtricarboxylic acid cycle (TCA) or Krebs cycle (named after its discoveror, Hans Adolf Krebs, the laureate of Nobel Prize in Physiology or Medicine 1953). In the TCA, there is a key process, which is also the only direct biochemical reaction generating high-energy phosphate bond, i. e. energy-rich thioester bond of succinyl-CoA is hydrolyzed by the catalysis of succinyl-CoA synthetase and coupled with the phosphorylation of guanosine diphosphate (GDP), resulting in generation of GTP. This is the metabolic process of generating energy of normal cells under the physiological condition of adequate oxygen supply (Figure 5), whereas cancer cells still choose another pathway called aerobic glycolysis to go even though they can acquire the same adequate oxygen supply as the normal cells. This phenomenon was discovered in 1924 by Otto Heinrich Warburg, the laureate of Nobel Prize in Physiology or Medicine 1931, so it is named Warburg effect (Figure 1-6). Although the Warburg effect was widely accepted by the scientists all over the world and the most advanced broad-spectrum clinical diagnostic equipment for cancer —positron emission computed tomography (PET) was developed based on the phenomenon, yet its underlying mechanism of biology and the significance-in-depth of clinical practice were still unclarified before. Why do cancer cells abandon the metabolic pathway of high-energy productivity (each molecule of consumed glucose produces 36-molecules ATP) and choose the low-energy one (each molecule of consumed glucose only produces 2-molecules ATP)?

Nearly a century has passed, the underlying meaning of this biological phenomenon is still a mystery puzzling scientists. Is it a fate or coincidence?

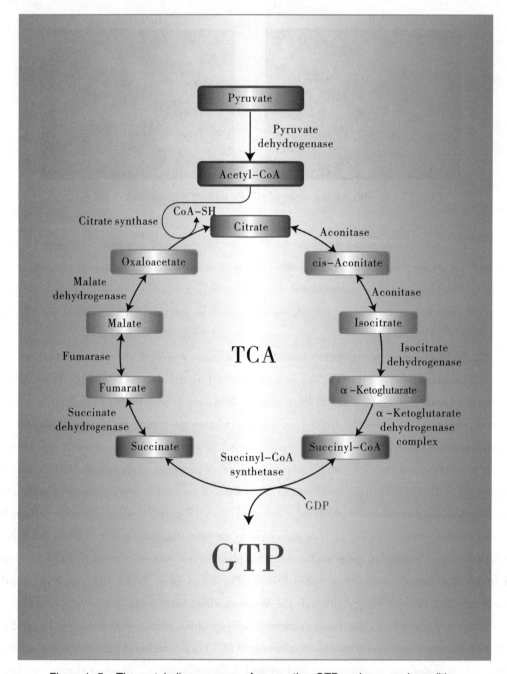

Figure 1-5　The metabolism process of generating GTP under normal condition

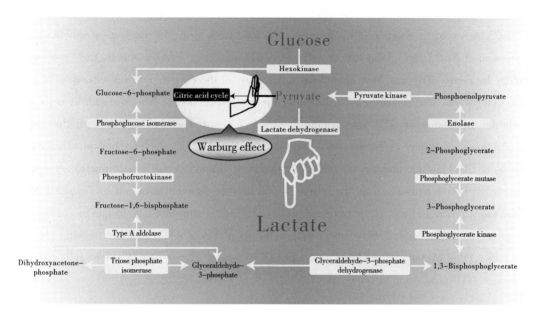

Figure 1-6   The warburg effect

By the clue of autostabilisis, we can find that cancer cells have to evade the metabolic pathway of TCA in order to survive. Talked above, the only step in the TCA to produce high-energy phosphate bonds at the substrate level is to generate GTP (Figure 1-5). Thus, cancer cells have to evade TCA by choosing the aerobic glycolysis to reduce GTP production. As the quantity of GTP decreases, the necessary raw materials for the assembly of microtubules will be insufficient, and then the assembly of microtubules will be reduced. Indeed, although its biological significance was not elucidated three decades ago, only half of the microtubules in various transformed cells, which stretch beneath the plasma membrane, were observed as compared with normal cells.

Microtubules are the source of generating the force causing nuclear compaction, so cancer cells can maintain that nuclear size is not drastically compacted during cell rounding by reducing GTP production, and so that cancer cells can evade the circompactosis and keep their malignant survival. Is there anything more important to organisms than survival? Isn't this the biological function and clinical significance-in-depth of Warburg effect, which has been eagerly sought for nearly a century!

When theinvestigation comes here, people may ask, is there any other way to generate GTP? Yes, it is ATP that transfers high-energy phosphate bonds to GDP, which is the second pathway to generate GTP. But this process has to be accomplished with the catalysis of nucleotide diphosphate kinase (NDPK), known as Nm23 (Figure 1-7). Surprisingly, *Nm*23 is the first discovered cancer cell metastasis suppressor gene. The expression of Nm23 was negatively correlated with the metastasis of various cancers and the survival of patients. Although the role of Nm23 in enzymatic reaction in biochemistry has long been clear, the mechanism why the high expression of Nm23 can inhibit cancer cell metastasis remains a mystery in cell-and-molecular biology for nearly 30 years. Now, according to the study of the catastrophic consequences of nuclear compaction, it is not difficult to find that the low expression of Nm23 in cancer cells inhibits the production of GTP from another pathway (Figure 1-8). Together with the aerobic glycolysis of cancer cells, the low expression of Nm23 joints the cell biological cascade process of blocking microtubule assembly. It reduces or eliminates the drastic nuclear compaction caused by microtubules from the source, which lays the foundation of cell-molecular biology for the survival and metastasis of cancer cells via evading autostabilisis. In fact, according to the principle of biochemical enzymatic reaction, the reduction of ATP caused by aerobic glycolysis (36 ATP of oxidative phosphorylation : 2 ATP of aerobic glycolysis) of cancer cells can also reduce GTP production to some extent.

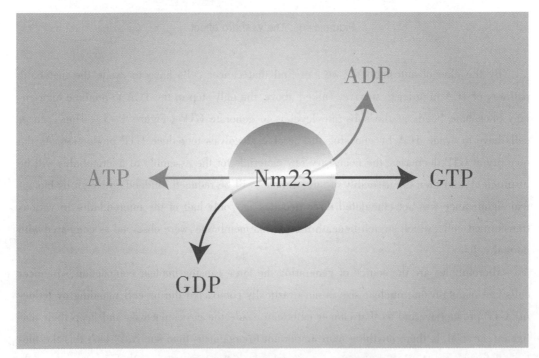

Figure 1-7 The catalytic action of Nm23

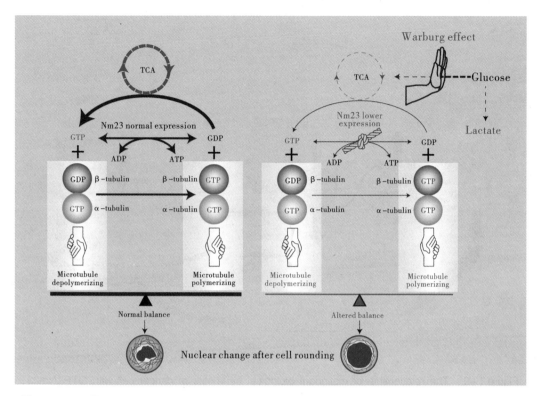

Figure 1-8　The effect of lower expression of Nm23 and aerobic glycolysis on polymerizing of microtubules

In summary, metabolic changes in GTP reduction, as a key factor, createthe notorious malignant biological behaviors of cancer cells that survive by evading circompactosis and lethal MIGI. Only by this way, can the cancer cells make invasive growth and distant metastasis possible (Figure 1-9).

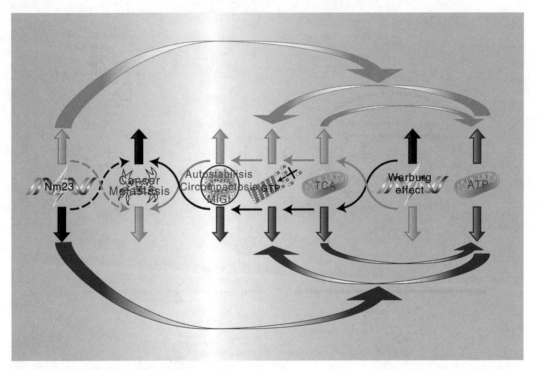

Figure 1-9   The relationship of malignant biological behaviors of cancer cell with GTP, Nm23, warburg effect and ATP

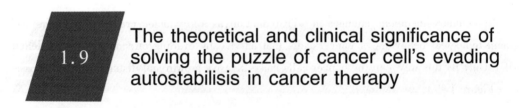

1.9   The theoretical and clinical significance of solving the puzzle of cancer cell's evading autostabilisis in cancer therapy

From the above investigation, it can be seen that circompactosis and lethal MIGI form the important autostabilic machinery evolved in maintaining the heredity and survival of advanced multicellular living beings. If cancer cells want to grow invasively and metastasize distantly, they have to evade circompactosis and lethal MIGI. Therefore, the reason why cancer cells choose the aerobic glycolysis pathway is that the metabolic mode is the most feasible, efficient and safe for cancer cells to evade circompactosis and lethal MIGI. Only in this way can the assembly of microtubules which can generate the nuclear-compaction force be restricted on a large scale without affecting the formation of microtubules which constitutes the normal structure of the spindle. In other words, the regulation of GTP quantity will only affect the large-scale production of microtubules, but will not cause the qualitative change of microtubules. Otherwise, for a cell, once the assembled microtubules undergoes hereditary structure changes, which seriously affect mitosis, its incidental consequences are ether lethality or genomic instability, and the ultimate consequences of frequent genetic damage will be fatal. Since the pathway of non-nuclear-compaction caused by the reduction of GTP and the assembly of microtubules is the key throat for the survival of cancer cells with malignant biological behaviors. If we can find the "Achilles heel" of the cancer cells according to their metabolic characteristics and implement fatal interventional measures, we can achieve the therapeutic effect of "locating the acupoint and sealing the throat with a sword" in accordance with the principle of "beating the snake seven inches" and killing the cancer cells. So where on earth are the dead spots of the cancer cells? We still need to follow the clue of nuclear compaction.

In order to evade GTP production pathway of TCA, cancer cells have to choose another alternative route, aerobic glycolysis. However, an important characteristic of aerobic glycolysis is that it produces a large amount of lactic acid. The Warburg effect revealed that the amount of glycolysis of cancer cells was 200 times higher than that of normal metabolic cells (this is the basis for the original invention of PET-CT, an important clinical high-tech applied in diagnoses of cancersfor their metastases). This means that cancer cells have to adopt corresponding levels of measures to expel the large amount of intracellular lactic acid, because the various biochemical reactions in human cells have very stringent physiological requirements for metabolic acid-base balance (near neutral). The consequences of lactic acid accumulation are serious. Clinical experience tells us that the consequences of lactic acidosis are fatal. Whereas, lactic acid efflux from cancer cells can not only evade intracellular acidosis, but also create conditions for their survival, invasion, diffusion and metastasis. Because the effect of efflux of lactic acid destroys the microenvironment of normal tissues, results in the death of normal cells and the destruction and degradation of extracellular matrix. According to the metabolic characteristics of the cancer cells, why can't we take advantage of their means of destroying normal tissues to "treat them in their own way", creating a counter-attack against their "Achilles heel"?

In ancient Chinese legend, there was a kind of divine beast named Pixiu. The magic is that Jade Emperor sealed its anus, that is, there is a mouth but no anus. Therefore, it can eat at will without expelling. Cancer cells, however, are not Jade Emperor's Pixiu. They devour a great deal of human nutrition throughout the day, and produce and drain a large amount of lactic acid to harm the normal human body. If we can block the "anus" of lactic acid efflux and let a large amount of lactic acid remain in the cancer cells themselves, can we achieve the specific therapeutic effect of killing cancer cells without harming normal tissues? Moreover, in the face of the large amount of lactic acid, even a small amount of blockade will lead to serious accumulation of lactic acid in the cancer cells. Just as for the torrential flood, if the discharge channel is not smooth, it will cause flooding. However, the same flood discharge conditions have little impact on the overall situation of the trickle flow. Then, what measures can we take to achieve this goal?

Firstly, we need is to find the "back door" of the cancer cell, which is the outlet of lactic acid. There is a protein family of monocarboxylate transporter (MCT) on the cell membrane. Among them, MCT4 is responsible for transporting the large amount of lactic acid produced by glycolysis to extracellular sites (Figure 1-10). In addition, there is a substance called proton pump on the cell membrane, which can pump hydrogen ions out of the cell. If we can block the main channels that maintain the acid-base balance in cancer cells, we will block the "back door" of large amount of lactic acid efflux from the cells, which will kill the cancer cells by the lethal acidosis of themselves. The cancer cells' life-gate was found, and the next was to find the blocking agents. We know that to develop a drug as a blocking agent, the cost is usually staggering (billions of dollars), the time is long (usually about 20 years), and the risk of failure is huge (usually 90%). Thanks to the gift of nature, "every cloud has a silver lining". As we know, there is a class of statins used to reduce blood-lipoids. One of the most serious side effects of these drugs is rhabdomyolysis. Why? Because striated muscle is the most important movement tissue of human body. In anaerobic conditions, the striated muscle undergoes glycolysis and produces a large amount of lactic acid. If the lactic acid cannot be excluded from the cells through MCT4, the lactic acid will be accumulated in the cells, and the striated muscle will be necrotized by dissolution. And statins are just the inhibitors of MCT4. Therefore, as long as we reasonably control the dosage of drugs according to the characteristics of cell lactic acid production higher than two orders of magnitude in normal tissues (Figure 1-11), and avoid inappropriate anaerobic exercise and hypoxic events in normal tissues, we can specifically kill cancer cells without harming normal tissues (Figure 1-10). Furthermore, in order to prevent cancer cells from escaping intracellular acidosis by proton pumping, we can use existing proton pump inhibitors, such as Omeprazole, to perform a second blockade (Figure 1-10). Also, in the treatment of diabetes, there is a kind of biguanide drugs. The most serious side effect of biguanides is lactic acidosis, which is also the reason why the early drugs such as phenethylbiguanide and butylbiguanide are discontinued. At present, the side effects of metformin on lactic acidosis are much lower than those of early biguanide drugs. However, the metformin still has the same pharmacological effect. Therefore, the use of metformin to increase the production of lactic acid can further improve the level of intracellular lactic acid accumulation leading to cell acidosis, constituting a synergistic killing of cancer cells (Figure 1-10). Because lactic acid produced at a reasonable dose has little effect on normal cells, but it is worse for cancer cells with higher lactic acid level. This is also the third lethal force on cancer cells. Furthermore, platelets play a key role in the adherent survival of cancer cells. To further block the "ganging, massing and clustering escape" and survival pathway of cancer cells, aspirin and/or warfarin were used to construct the fourth lethal killer of cancer cells. Under the action of these drugs, the cancer cells with aggressive, rapid growth and distant metastasis of malignant phenotypes will be suppressed.

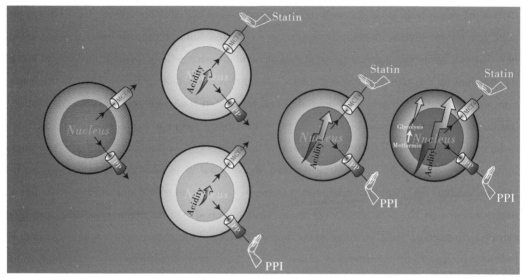

Figure 1-10   Schematic of blocking-acid-gate therapy specific to cancer

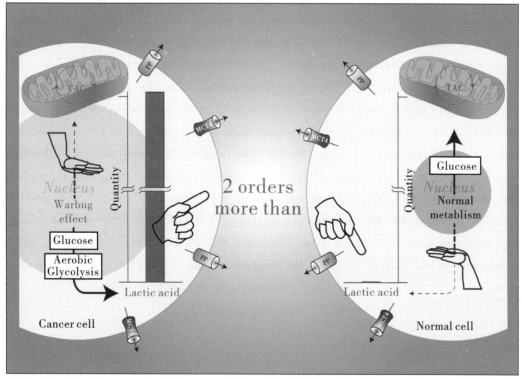

Figure 1-11   The contrast of Warburg effect and production of lactate between cancer and normal cells

If cancer cells do not take the aerobic glycolysis route, what will happen? Cancer tissue is a highly heterogeneous cell population. When the cancer cell population with malignant biological behaviors such as rapid invasive growth and metastasis is controlled and killed, some cancer tissues may have residual of the well differentiated cancer cell subpopulations that have not entered the aerobic glycolysis pathway. The cancer cells that survive through heterogeneous selection can only grow in a mode similar to that of normal tissue cells or benign tumors, and are either tolerant or resistant to conventional radiotherapy and chemotherapy. In view of this situation, we can treat the tumors with beheaded and eradicated treatment such as surgery, ablation, intratumoral injection and other means as far as possible. Of course, for tumors that are difficult to be completely removed at one time, surgical measures can be taken to minimize the tumor burden. Then, through the above drug regimen, the original state of invasive cancer can be reconstructed into the boundary relationship between cancer tissue and normal tissue similar to benign tumors. By this way, a new operation window period can be created, and the operation can be performed again. This is based on the fact that the drug regimen plays a key role in controlling the spread and metastasis of cancer cells. Under these conditions, a new concept of operation indications can be established, which follows the treatment regimen similar to that for benign tumors, but involves the removal of metastatic lesions. Because, firstly, the cancer cells do not grow in an invasive and metastatic way at this time; secondly, this drug regimen can prevent the metastasis of cancer cells during perioperative period. To say the least, if cancer cells break through their growth patterns similar to benign tumors via genetic mutations (such as MIGI) or epigenetic pathway, they can only go to the pathway of aerobic glycolysis, which is just the target of this drug regimen. Otherwise, if the rounded cancer cells do not attempt to metastasize distantly through aerobic glycolysis pathway, their destiny will only be natural senescence and death (including circompactosis). Even if some cancer cells become the "fishes that leak out of the net", it will gain time and lay a foundation for the implementation of comprehensive measures to cure cancer with such a wide range of systemic drugs and various surgical operations. Of course, any treatment has its indications and contraindications, that is to say, no matter what kind of treatment is not omnipotent, this kind of BAG method which makes cancer cells' acidic death is the same. The inappropriate use of this method will be described below.

The spectrum of cancers suitable for therapy with BAG regimen

No matter what kind of cells, including the cells of solid tissues and blood system, and whatever genetic mutations or epigenetic changesthat the cells depend on, they have to fulfill an important prerequisite if they want to break through the normal tissue structure and develop into cancers that grow invasively and metastasize distantly through the circulatory system. That is to say, only by resisting circompactosis and lethal MIGI can these cells survive through evading autostabilisis in the course of metastasis and in the state of invasion, and then the malignant biological behaviors of invasion and metastasis can be realized. Therefore, in theory, the therapeutic strategy for Warburg effect is suitable for the rapid growth, invasion and metastasis of all cancers (including solid-tumor-type cancers and blood-system cancers leukemia).

Therapeutic strategies for solid cancer

Surgical radical resection of cancer tissue is worldwide recognized as the only therapy for solid tumors that can be eradicated. However, it is regrettable that the cancers of many patients have developed to a stage where the existing surgical methods can not completely remove them; or, the cancer cells have metastasized far away, but the current technology can not detect them. Even if the primary lesion is resected by surgery, its subclinical metastases will quickly develop into clinical metastases. Or, because of the complexity of surgery and the limitations of technology, the operation inevitably results in the dissemination of cancer cells; in addition, the malignant growth of cancer has caused diffuse involvement of important organs. In these cases, the feasibility, significance and effect of the operation will be questioned by traditional evaluation. The focus of the problem is undoubtedly the limitations of surgery. Ultimately, it is also the root cause of malignant tumors: invasion and metastasis, because it is the culprit of cancer's untreatable and lethal nature. However, the systematic therapies investgated in this study are based on the premise of specifically targeting the invasive growth and distant metastasis of cancer cells. The main effects of this systematic therapy are included as follows: ① Cancers whose metabolism is in the mode of high glycolysis can be killed. ② For the cancers suitable for immediate operation, the therapy can kill high metastatic cancer cells before and after operation, so as to avoid the possible metastasis caused by operation. ③ For cancers unsuitable for immediate surgery, invasive and potentially distant metastatic cancer cells can be killed first, and the heterogeneous cancers can be reconstructed into tumors similar to benign tumor growth patterns, so that a suitable window can be created to perform the operation. ④ According to the current treatment criteria, patients who have lost operation significance can be treated by killing invasive and possibly distant metastatic cancer cells, preventing distant metastasis of primary lesion and re-metastasis of secondary lesions, and reconstructing heterogeneous cancer cells in primary and secondary lesions into a growth mode similar to benign tumors, so as to create a therapeutic window with operative significance. ⑤ For patients with high recurrence tendency after operation, preventive treatment with this regimen can be used to kill dormant cancer cells and prevent their recurrence and metastasis. The reason why this therapeutic goal can be achieved is that the regimen can specifically target the metabolic characteristics of dormant cancer cells with aerobic glycolysis mode, and the characteristics of distant metastasis after the release of dormant state. ⑥ For brain metastases, the regimen can be administered through the blood-brain barrier to kill cancer cells and/or create a surgical window. ⑦ Cancers that are not suitably treated by surgery can be treated with the regimen to kill cancer cells (such as small-cell cancer, large-cell cancer, etc.) that grow all over the body. ⑧ This regimen can alleviate tissue-lactate-accumulation and non-nerve-injury cancer-pain caused by the excretion of lactic acid from cancer cells.

1.12 Therapeutic strategies for leukemia

Leukemia is a kind of systemic malignant tumors, originating from hematopoietic tissue of malignant transformation. The pathogenic characteristics of leukemia are abnormal proliferation of malignant hematopoietic cells, destruction of hematopoietic tissue, loss of normal hematopoietic function of hematopoietic tissue, and invasion of important organs of the whole body by cancer cells, resulting in severe fatal lesions such as anemia, hemorrhage, decreased immunity, organ failure, brain and nervous system injury. Therefore, the therapeutic goal of leukemia is to kill leukemic cells and restore, rebuild and maintain normal hematopoietic function. Although there are many treatment measures for leukemia, such as radiotherapy, induction of differentiation, immunity, hematopoietic stem cell transplantation and so on, the conventional chemotherapeutics to kill leukemic cells are still the most basic and important therapies in clinic.

Especially for acute leukemia, only by quickly and effectively controlling and killing large-scale proliferation of leukemic cells, can we save the lives of patients, create conditions for follow-up treatment, that is, make follow-up therapy possible. However, conventional chemotherapy and other means of killing leukemic cells can produce serious toxic and side effects, including bone marrow suppression, tissue and functional damage of liver and kidney andother important organs, immune suppression, severe gastrointestinal side-effects, infection and so on. And periodic chemotherapy is easy to induce the drug resistance of leukemic cells. Moreover, the high cost of leukemia treatment is a heavy financial burden to patients and their families, as well as to society. In addition, even if the treatment cost for refractory leukemic patients is high (including the tremendous mental and physical pain caused by the treatment and the extremely bad quality of life), the current treatment methods are still helpless and can not save the lives of patients.

So, is there a treatment method that can overcome or reduce the serious side effects of the existing treatment methods on leukemic patients and improve the cure rate of patients on the premise of alleviating the pain of patients, improving the quality of patients' life? This is still to be investigated from the most basically cellular and molecular biologic and histopathologic characteristics of leukemia. Although leukemia is a systemic hematopoietic tissue lesion, and the lesion can invade the whole body organs, its initial onset does not originate from the whole body hematopoietic tissue at the same time. Because of the histological characteristics of the blood system, there is no obvious change in peripheral blood and no clinical manifestation in the initial stage of the disease, so it is difficult to find the initial pathological changes of patients. Once a patient is diagnosed due to clinical symptoms, the lesion often affects the whole body hematopoietic tissue or other organs. The stage of the disease is far from the initial lesion, so there will be no "cancer in situ" concept of solid cancer for leukemia. The reason why leukemia can develop into a malignant phenotype of systemic hematopoietic tissue lesion and systemic organ invasion is that the metabolic of leukemic cells has transformed into a mode dominated by aerobic glycolysis. This is true for both lymphoid and myeloid leukemia. However, it is just because of this change in metabolic pattern that it lays the foundation for killing leukemia cells by the drugs causing intracellular acidosis (blocking-acid-gate therapy, BAG). And the characteristics of this metabolic model naturally endow the corresponding BAG regimen with specificity for the cancer cell therapy. The drugs used in the regimen can overcome the side effects of conventional chemotherapy and other killing methods with serious toxicity. In addition, the administration mode is simple, which provides great convenience for the treatment. Moreover, the low cost of the drug treatment can reduce enormous economic and social burdens for patients and society, and help millions of patients and families get rid of the predicament of leukemia.

1.13　Attentions in the therapy

Firstly, treatment must be carried out strictly and normatively under the guidance of professional doctors.

Any drug entering the human bodyhas to metabolize and expel its residual and harmful metabolites through the corresponding tissues and organs. Otherwise it will cause the accumulation and poisoning of the corresponding substances. The drugs used in this regimen also need corresponding metabolism, so the regimen also has its strict scope and rules of treatment for adaptive diseases. Therefore, in addition to the relevant taboos stipulated in the Pharmacopoeia and the drug instructions, the following items are particularly important in the application of this regimen in the treatment of cancer patients, and must be noted.

Whether for cancer patients or non-cancer patients, functional failure of vital organs is the direct cause of death. Once the patient suffers from acute organ failure, if it can not be effectively treated and improved, the patient's condition will deteriorate drastically, leading to rapid death of the patient. In contrast, the treatment of cancer is a relatively slow process. Therefore, for organ damage and dysfunction and failure of important organs caused by any reason, appropriate treatment measures should be taken to restore their basic functions before the regimen can be used for treatment.

Important organ damage mainly includes: ①Liver, kidney, heart, lung (including pulmonary fibrosis, hypoxemia, etc.) dysfunction and failure caused by toxic and side effects of chemical drugs (including the drugs in chemotherapeutics, targeting therapy, analgesics, and etc.), radiation damage, and toxic and side effects of biotherapy (such as various cell- and immune-therapy). ②Severe bone marrow suppression caused by toxic side effects of chemical drugs and radiation damage, and extensive bone marrow destruction caused by cancer metastasis, resulting in loss of hematopoietic function, etc. ③Gastrointestinal obstruction (including esophagus, biliary tract, intestine, etc.). For such patients, only after the corresponding surgery (such as stent placement, fistula, etc.) treatment, obstruction has been relieved, and then the regimen can be used as appropriate according to the changes of patient's condition. ④Severe organ damage, systemic multiple organ failure due to tumor invasion in advanced and end-stage patients, and inability to eat.

In addition, attention should be paid to the following treatmentissues: ①In the course of treatment, avoid anaerobic exercise, avoid the occurrence of systemic and local ischemia, hypoxia and circulatory impairment. ②For children under 10 years of age and pregnant women, it is not appropriate to use the drugs until the side effects of the regimen are clear. ③Strict attention should be paid to the possible side effects of long-term use of proton pump inhibitors such as omeprazole, and the rational use of the drugs is necessary. ④In theory, metformin and aspirin are double-edged swords. They have different effects at different stages of cancer, that is, they can promote the evolution and development of cancer cells or kill cancer cells according to different cellular states. Therefore, rational combination therapy should be selected to overcome the shortcomings of single drug and improve the curative effect. ⑤When a large number of cancer tissues excreting lactic acid and causing cancer pain are quickly destroyed by this therapy, the cancer pain caused by the lactic acid will be relieved. At this time, if large doses of addictive analgesics used before are stopping, the drug withdrawal symptoms will occur. The corresponding treatment needs consultation with related disciplines.

In conclusion, BAG therapy is characterized by killing highly invasive and metastatic cancer cells(solid tumor and leukemia) with aerobic glycolysis as the main metabolic mode; specifically preventing primary and secondary metastases of cancer; killing dormant cancer cells to prevent their recurrence and metastasis; creating a new surgical window period for the residual cancers, which are remodeled into the tissue structure similar to benign tumor after the cancer cells with the main metabolic mode of aerobic glycolysis as well as highly invasive and metastatic natures have been killed, and relieving the non-nerve-injured cancer pain caused by lactic acid efflux from cancer cells and its accumulation in tissues; in addition to the therapeutic characteristics stated above, this drug therapeutic regimen also has the characteristics of not easy to produce drug-resistance and maintaining high quality of life of patients.

Chapter 2

▶ Solving a Series of Biological and Medical Puzzles

2.1   What is the safety bottleneck in stem cell therapy (can the therapy cause gene mutation and carcinogenesis)

With the discovery of stem cells, people place unlimited expectations on their application, hoping to use stem cells to treat many diseases. Although hematopoietic stem cell transplantation has been more mature in clinical application. However, the ruthless reality is that the application of embryonic stem cell (ESC), induced–pluripotent stem cell (iPS), and somatic committed stem cell (CSC) is not easy. It has been recognized that embryonic stem cells and induced pluripotent stem cells are tumorigenic, that is, embryonic stem cells implanted into the body will form a mixed embryonic tumor, teratoma. Therefore, it is envisaged that embryonic stem cells can be differentiated into specific tissue cells by induced differentiation and then used for corresponding treatment to avoid the risk of tumorigenesis in embryonic stem cell therapy. Therefore, people have focused on how to purify differentiated cells, that is, how to remove undifferentiated embryonic stem cells from differentiated cells for treatment. At the same time, it is speculated that another risk factor for iPS treatment comes from exogenous inducible factors. Therefore, how to optimize the inducible factors of iPS has become a research hotspot to avoid the risk of stem cell therapy. From this point of view, a lot of work has been done, including clinical trial. For example, Japan has implemented the first stem cell therapy for patients with retinal degeneration. However, the anticipated treatment of the second case of retinal degeneration was discontinued because of the discovery of risky genetic mutations in the cells expected for treatment. This clinical example demonstrates that in the absence of a clear understanding of the cause of genetic mutations involved in the stem cell therapy, the risk and catastrophe of stem cell therapy can only be assessed by blind tentative and guessing, and the risk can not be avoided scientifically, so it is difficult to control how to obtain safe therapeutic cells. The clinical safety of stem cell therapy can only be reasonably guaranteed if clinical trials are based on mature theories to elucidate the mechanism of gene mutation in stem cell therapy. The primary aim of stem cell therapy is to obtain enough cellsthat can perform normal physiological functions to repair, reconstruct or replace the lesion tissues and organs. Therefore, obtaining a sufficient number of normal cells for treatment is a prerequisite for stem cell therapy. Moreover, the specific functions of various tissues and organs are based on the cells' corresponding differentiation. Without differentiated cells, there is no physiological function of tissues and organs. So the focus of stem cell therapy is cellular differentiation. Since embryonic stem cells and induced pluripotent stem cells have tumorigenic (teratoma) problems that prevent them from being directly implanted into the body, is it safe to implant committed stem cells and differentiated cells into the body? To answer this question, we have to go back to the process of stem cell therapy.

Embryonic stem cells are undifferentiated cells formed at a specific time and location space in the early embryonic stage, which do not exist in normal adults. Whereas, the iPS is a kind of pluripotent stem cell formed by inducing the differentiated somatic cells through exogenous factors, which does not exist in normal body. Because embryonic stem cells have strict requirements on the environmental signal program and the time program of differentiation, any disorder of the programs will bring serious consequences. The artificial teratoma is the result of the implantation of embryonic stem cells in the wrong time, place and space. Therefore, in order to obtain sufficient number of differentiated cells for treatment through embryonic stem cells, the expansion in vitro is the conventional measures. However, in order to maintain their own stability, advanced multicellular living beings have established a rigorous machinery of autostabilisis. The complete functional system of this autostabilic machinery exists in each normal cell itself, and the natural law endows each normal cell with the need to enter the pathway of apoptosis in the condition of non-physiological cell rounding through this autostabilic machinery, in order to maintain the overall safety of the body. Therefore, both in vivo and in vitro, the differentiated somatic cells of advanced multicellular living beings adhere to the inherent characteristics of autostabilisis, that is, once embryonic stem cells are differentiated, both committed stem cells and differentiated cells are strictly controlled by the machinery of autostabilisis. Cell spreading, growth factors, and accessibility-control-mechanisms of growth factors (such as the occluding structure of tight junction and the molecular control of basement membrane) constitute the basic central mechanisms in the regulation of normal proliferation of somatic cells. Furthermore, in order to avoid cell's escaping from the restriction of these basic proliferation-control links under the circumstance of cell rounding, the advanced living beings have further formed their inherent autostabilic machinery based on circompactosis and lethal MIGI, thus restricting the normal cells' proliferation and ectopic plantation similar to malignant cancer cells. It is worth noting that once normal cells become rounded (Figure 2-1) due to non-physiological factors, even if they can escape circompactosis by re-spreading, the loss of protection of the single-stranded DNA chains by losing their binding proteins (RPA, POT1), which constitutes the important molecular basis of MIGI, will prevent them from escaping the catastrophic fate of MIGI (Figure 2-1). More importantly, no matter for embryonic stem cells, induced pluripotent stem cells, mesenchymal stem cells or umbilical cord blood stem cells, as long as there are in vitro processes involved in the acquisition, induction of dedifferentiation and/or re-differentiation, and culture and expansion of the cells, the occurrence of cell rounding will not be avoided. Therefore, if these differentiated cells to be used for stem cell therapy have to undergo the in vitro treatment, they will not escape the fate of circompactosis and MIGI. The latter includes senescence, tumorigenesis, and the risk of large-scale gene mutation. At present, due to the lack of non-invasive safety-risk-detection methods of examining every differentiated cell to be used for stem cell therapy, the safety-risk assessment of cell therapy can only be inferred by gene mutation and latent risk of mutant cells in cell population, and pathogenic exposure within limited observation time after treatment. However, the short-term non-exposure of the disease can not exclude the long-term safety risks. Therefore, the "latency" of pathogenicity in the subsequent evolution of genetic variation is undoubtedly a high risk factor for therapeutic safety. This risk of MIGI naturally poses a safety bottleneck for stem cell therapy. How to break through this safety bottleneck is a formidable challenge to stem cell therapy (Figure 2-1).

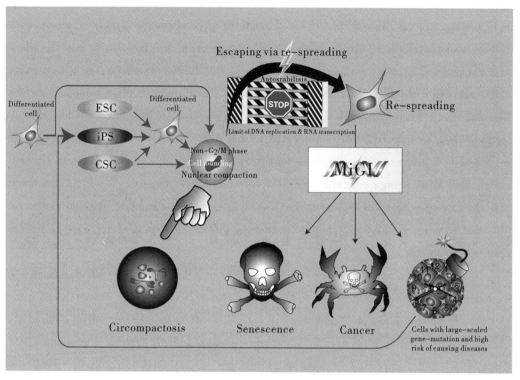

Figure 2-1 The fate of stem cells manipulated by in vitro treatment related to cellular differentiation

2.2 Are cancer cells characterized by genomic stability or genomic instability

Gene mutation caused by genomic instability is an important cause of tumorigenesis (excluding the direct effects of chemical and biological mutagenic carcinogenic actors, and ultraviolet and radiation irradiation). This has become the consensus of decades of long-term research in cancer field. However, what are the states of genomic stability of cancerous cells? In other words, is the genome of a cancer cell stable or unstable? This question has been an important and controversial puzzle. How to elucidate this problem from the mechanism is very important for understanding the occurrence and development of cancer and formulating correct clinical treatment strategies and regimens. The experiments about MIGI suggest that genomic instability based on MIGI principles is a key factor in carcinogenesis. Once cancer cells are formed, their growth pattern, MIGI-based genomic state and the metabolic pattern are inevitably coupled, that is, there are two types of growth, metabolism and genomic stability patterns. One type is that cancer cells stabilize their genomes through the mode of aerobic glycolysis, which also evades circompactosis and MIGI. At this time, cancer cells can grow in a fast, disordered and malignant biological way, getting rid of the autostabilisis. Another type is that cancer cells grow and proliferate under the control of autostabilisis, which is close to normal metabolism and controlled by circompactosis. Once cells are rounded, their genome will lose the protection of single-stranded DNA-binding proteins and enters MIGI state. Therefore, the cells can only grow in a manner similar to benign tumors. Otherwise, the fate of circompactosis, immediately-lethal MIGI, aging death, non-immediately-lethal MIGI (large-scale genetic variation), and epigenetic changes will be inevitable. Of course, cancer cells similar to benign tumors can also evolve their metabolic patterns into the former through non-immediately-lethal MIGI or epigenetic pathways.

In any case, the goal of cancer cell evolution is to adapt and survive. If the purpose of evolution is to perish, will there be continued evolution? If the genome cannot adapt to the new growth mode of rapid proliferation out of control, resulting in frequent MIGI-induced stochastic and large-scale gene mutations, the consequences will be fatal. On the contrary, only when cancer cells adapt to new ways of growth and survival and maintain the stability of their genomes can they continue to proliferate and survive steadily in the way of maintaining their malignant biological behavior, such as invasion, diffusion and metastasis. Therefore, no matter what genetic changes, if cancer cells want to grow in the way of malignant biological behavior, they have to take the metabolic pathway of aerobic glycolysis to evade the lethal effects of circompactosis and MIGI. Under this condition, the genome naturally tends to be stable. HeLa cells are the most typical representative. This cell line has survived for nearly 70 years since it was removed from the cervical cancer tissue of American women (Henrietta Lacks) in 1951. It has been cultured, reproduced, and passaged in countless laboratories all over the world. It has become an important tool for biomedical study such as cancer research. Five Nobel Prizes have been awarded for research related to HeLa cells. The greatness of this cell line lies not only in the fact that it has played an important role in the cause of human health, but also in the fact that its magic is and will bring us more enlightenment in understanding the nature of life and cancer. Although HeLa cells have multiplied more than 50 million tons so far, equivalent to more than 100 Empire State Buildings in New York, their genomes are very stable. In 2013, studies found that HeLa cells exhibit remarkable genomic stability even in point mutations. Undoubtedly, this cancer cell line with typical malignant biological behaviors has also given us a crucial hint on the mechanism of stable survival by evading MIGI and circompactosis through altering its metabolic pattern.

2.3　Why does inflammation cause cancer

Not everyone will be exposed to carcinogenic doses of mutagens and radiation in their lifetime, but few people have experienced any kind of inflammation in their lifetime, including biological inflammation (such as respiratory tract infections caused by colds, as well as lung, liver, kidney, stomach, intestine, brain, nose, pharynx, mouth, limbs, skin and other biological infectious inflammation), physical inflammation (such as traumatic inflammation, which can be open and non-open), chemical inflammation (such as drug-induced inflammation), and mixed inflammation (such as physical, chemical combined with biological infection, etc.). In addition to the common features of inflammation – red, swollen, hot and painful, another important feature of inflammation is cell rounding and exfoliation, which is caused by the changes of tissue structure in the inflammation site. Therefore, exfoliative cytology is a very important subject on which clinical medical practice depends. It can complement pathology at the cellular level and provide the most direct and authoritative basis for clinical diagnosis. In addition to the significance of cell rounding and exfoliation, a common event in advanced living beings, in diagnostics, the MIGI as a deep factor of this event also provides clues for us to understand why inflammation cause cancer from the cellular and molecular biological level. Therefore, it is clear that inflammation and injury are sources of MIGI, which has important clinical significance for us to actively prevent and treat inflammation, especially for defensive intervening the recurrence of cell rounding and re-spread caused by repeated chronic inflammation.

2.4　What is cancer stem cell, what is the relationship between so-called "cancer stem cells" and cancer treatment

Cancer stem cells are now believed to be responsible for cancer metastasis, recurrence and tolerance to radiotherapy and chemotherapy. One of the most important concepts in the definition of so-called "cancer stem cells" is infinite proliferation. This ability is undoubtedly the basis of metastasis of cancer cells. However, how to use this concept to explain drug resistance and relapse is not very clear. Except the cancer cells' drug-resistance that is acquired or induced by repeated chemotherapy, the regularity of initial resistance of cancer cells in vivo to radiotherapy and chemotherapy is that the cells with lower proliferation level and well-differentiation state are more tolerant to radiotherapy and chemotherapy; on the contrary, the cells with more active proliferation and poor-differentiation state are more sensitive to radiotherapy and chemotherapy. This is why chemotherapy and radiotherapy are prone to cause bone marrow suppression, alopecia, mucosal ulcer and other tissue damage with rich committed stem cells of rapid proliferation and renewal. However, the so-called "cancer stem cells" not only have high proliferation activity similar to committed stem cells, but also have aerobic glycolysis similar to embryonic stem cells. This enables cancer stem cells to acquire the characteristics of dormancy under harsh living microenvironment, which is one of the most difficult states to treat in clinic. Furthermore, cancer cells can undergo a "stubborn dedifferentiation" transformation, which is different from embryonic stem cells, due to genetic variation of genes. They can also undergo metabolic transformation due to epigenetic changes, and thus acquire stemness. However, according to the characteristics of epigenetic reversibility, the cancer cells with the stemness acquired by epigenetic changes can still change back to the metabolic pattern similar to that of benign tumors, which provides a theoretical basis and guiding principles for the accurate assessment of therapeutic outcomes and the dynamic design of therapeutic regimens. So "cancer stem cells" is actually a vague concept. Generally speaking, all the cancer cells that can form lethal metastatic cancer should belong to the so-called "cancer stem cells". If lethal metastasis is abandoned, the so-called "cancer stem cells" will lose their meaning. The so-called stem has the main connotation of "origin". A lethal metastatic cancer can originate directly from cancer cells with highly malignant biological behaviors (rapid proliferation, invasive growth, distant metastasis, etc.) or from cancer cells that have not escaped the limitation of autostabilisis (MIGI and circompactosis), although the process of carcinogenesis has been completed (the minimum number of mutations of oncogenes or tumor suppressor genes required for carcinogenesis). Although the latter does not have the malignant biological behaviors of the former for the time being, it has the possibility of mutating into the former at any time through the action of MIGI and other factors causing gene mutation and epigenetic changes. Therefore, the stemness of the former is undeniable, while the latter can naturally acquire lethal stemness by crossing the apoptotic and senescent pathways of circompactosis and MIGI through metabolic changes and stepping into the malignant pathway of anti-autostabilic immortalization. That is to say, so-called "cancer stem cells" can be transformed from so-called "non-stemness" cancer cells at any time. The latter is more resistant to radiotherapy, chemotherapy and immunotherapy. Therefore, the research and design of prevention and treatment strategies to deal with the latter's stemness development, evolution-related events and consequences are the key to cure cancer or to achieve "cancer-bearing" survival. This is an important reason why the concepts (autostabilisis, MIGI and circompactosis) developed in this study have been successfully used to guide clinical practice.

2.5   Why can cancer cells be dormant

Recurrence is an important cause of cancer's being a refractory disease. We have investigated the so-called "cancer stem cells" for cancer recurrence. In fact, exploring the so-called "cancer stem cells" has to involve another important concept – dormancy. When cancer cells enter a state of "sleep" or quiescence, which neither proliferates nor dies, due to changes in some environmental factors, the so-called dormancy is formed. Why can cancer cells "sleep"? Microenvironment destruction and remodeling caused by treatment, inflammation, cancer growth and other factors can lead to changes in the relationship among cancer cells, their adjacent cells and extracellular matrix. The remodeled extracellular matrix can encapsulate cancer cells. As investigated in the previous paragraph, extracellular matrix (ECM) has permeability and accessibility-limiting effects on growth factors dependent on cell proliferation. At this time, cancer cells can enter a dormant state if the survival environment fulfills the following conditions. ① The structure of extracellular matrix reached the state of allowing small nutrients to penetrate and restricting protein-like growth factors. ② The number of cancer cells is small, which can reduce the consumption of nutrients and ensure that the consumption of nutrients matches the infiltration rate; and the harmful substances of cell efflux are less and easy to dissipate (such as lactic acid) so as not to have serious destructive effects on the microenvironment. ③ Proliferation of cancer cells have to depend on growth factors from routine sources (without autocrine of growth factors). ④ No abnormal growth factor signaling pathway (including gene mutation) was activated. ⑤ Aerobic glycolysis is the main energy metabolism. Once the dormant environment and state of cancer cells caused by the above conditions are destroyed by inflammation and injury such as the events of biology, physics and chemistry, cancer cells will be like hungry beasts after dormancy, preying and expanding crazily, thus forming fatal cancer recurrence and metastasis. Although this kind of dormant cancer cells will be resistant to radiotherapy and chemotherapy due to the inductive effect of long-term treatment and the limitation of the maximum treatment doses, even no effect for cellular immunotherapy on the dormant cancer cells, yet theoretically speaking, the regimen introduced above can play a therapeutic role in killing this kind of dormant cancer cells and put these latent cancer cells to death.

2.6 How do advanced multicellular living beings construct natural defense mechanism, what is its clinical significance in cancer prevention and treatment

If advanced multicellular living beings want to survive, they need to construct their natural defense mechanism to maintain the safety of their own survival. So what are the main natural risks to the survival of advanced multicellular living beings? Two aspects are the most basic: exogenous-pathogenic-factors invasion and endogenous-abnormal cell growth. Firstly, in order to remove invasive primary pathogens and the consequently secondary pathogens resulting in tissue damage, the body has evolved the defensive immune machinery (Immunity) (Figure 2-2). Furthermore, in order to maintain normal tissue structure, avoid and prevent the abnormal growth of rounded and exfoliated cells caused by tissue damage, the body has evolved the autostabilic machinery (Figure 2-2). That is to say, the autostabilic machinery that functions through nuclear compaction based on mitochondria, microtubules, "Junk" DNA (non-coding DNA) and nuclei as core elements is unique to the cells of advanced multicellular living beings. Compared with lower single-cell organisms, the autostabilic machinery laid down by circompactosis and lethal MIGI of somatic cells is the foundation of forming advanced multicellular living beings. The reason why autostabilisis becomes the lifeline of advanced multicellular living beings is that the characteristics of exfoliation and metabolism of advanced multicellular living beings determine that the life process of advanced multicellular living beings depends on the metabolic renewal of cells (from proliferation and differentiation to senescence and exfoliation). This kind of cell metabolism has to be based on maintaining a strict physiological structure, because only by maintaining a strict physiological structure, various tissues and organs can exercise their normal physiological functions. However, in the natural state, the cells of advanced multicellular biological tissues and organs will be invaded by non-physiological pathogenic factors all the time, so it will inevitably cause the pathological cell-rounding and exfoliation of cells. In order to avoid the tissue destruction of physiological structure caused by non-physiological planting growth of exfoliated cells, the organisms have evolved the autostabilic machinery consisting of circompactosis, lethal MIGI and adhesion selection (such as tissue-specific selection of integrin and other adhesion molecule families). With this autostabilic machinery, advanced multicellular living beings can prevent the crazy growth of exfoliated cells (including normal cells, benign tumor cells and malignant tumor cells similar to benign tumors), thus avoiding the loss of physiological function of tissues and organs. Otherwise, non-physiological exfoliated normal cells, like invasive and metastatic cancer cells, will grow wantonly in a malignant biological way, turning the body into a confused mass of uncontrolled cells with no or disordered physiological function. However, without the organs and systems functioning physiologically, advanced multicellular living beings cannot survive.

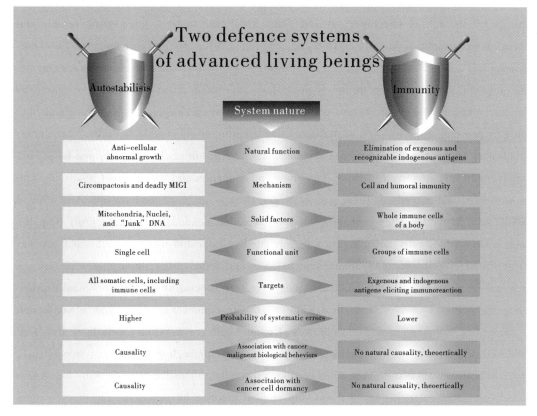

Figure 2-2　Main characteristics of the two natural defense systems for advanced living beings

Since the whole body cells are restricted by the machinery ofautostabilisis, the immune cells, which are part of the body and determine the function of the immune system, are also naturally restricted by this machinery. For solid tissue cells, if their genetic system is in the abnormal state making aerobic glycolysis be main metabolic mode, the cells will escape the limitation of autostabilisis to produce solid tumors with malignant biological behaviors. If immune cells escape the limitation of autostabilisis through abnormal metabolic change, they will also develop into hematological cancer—leukemia. In addition to the carcinogenesis of immune cells themselves, the immune mechanism has an important relationship with the occurrence of solid tumors induced by the tissue damage caused and external pathogenic invasion. When external inflammation-causing pathogens invade the body, they will not only cause inflammatory tissue damage, but also causing a previously neglected event, that is, somatic cell rounding. Although completely exfoliated cells with normal metabolism are difficult to escape from the fate of circompactosis, the rounded cells in situ facing circompactosis are more likely to obtain the chance of "reborn" which can avoid death but bring a latent disaster, carcinogenesis, to the body. Because, as long as the rounded cells can re-spread before the opening of circompactosis, they will escape the role of circompactosis and lethal MIGI, and undergo large-scale genetic and chromosomal mutations due to the effects of non-lethal MIGI, laying the foundation for cainogenesis and aging. Therefore, even if there are two sets of natural defense machinery, immunity and autostabilisis, to maintain the safety of the body, the tissue inflammatory damage caused by various pathogenic factors is still an unavoidable important carcinogenic event throughout life. Only by preventing the invasion of pathogens and avoiding or eliminating the role of various inflammatory factors can the occurrence of inflammatory tissue-injury be reduced; and by active, timely, rapid and effective treatment, the chronic inflammation and its persistent recurrence can be prevented and minimized. These preventive and therapeutic measures have important clinical significance in reducing the probability of gene mutation needed for carcinogenesis from the source. More importantly, according to the elucidated cellular and molecular biological mechanism of cancer cells' escaping from circompactosis and lethal MIGI through genetic changes in metabolic patterns, a new therapeutic strategy has been successfully tested in clinical practice under the guidance of these theoretical concepts. The first pioneering therapeutic breakthrough in preventing malignant biological behaviors of cancer cells, invasion and metastasis, has been achieved. Moreover, it has the characteristics of high specificity, low toxicity and side effects, low cost of drugs and convenient administration. Especially, this method also lays the foundation of cell-and-molecular-biological theory and clinical practice for prolonging the life of cancer patients and improving the cure rate of cancer on the premise of maintaining patients' high quality of life.

2.7 Is somatic cell cloning safe

Many years ago, people began to clone animals with somatic cells in order to do some ideal things. However, there has been a lack of theoretical clarification on the safety of somatic cell cloning. This study suggests that under the operation of existing methods and techniques, a large -scale gene mutation can be caused by MIGI in a single passage of normal somatic cells, which may be one of the reasons why somatic cell cloning is difficult to succeed. Moreover, even if such cloning escapes lethal gene mutations, its stochastic and MIGI – induced large – scale gene mutations will not make the cloned off spring have the same genes and phenotypes, and large–scale gene mutations is like a time bomb, laying a catastrophic genetic risk for future follow–up diseases. Dolly, a somatic cell clone sheep born 22 years ago, may still be remembered for her euthanasia due to sickly constitution, and has brought some useful and vital warning to people.

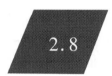

2.8   Why do cancer patients quickly lose weight and develop cachexia

The so–called "cachexia" refers to a pathological state in which cancer patients are extremely emaciated and suffer from systemic physiological – function disorders. The malignant consumption of cancer tissue is the most serious cause. In malignant cancer cells, the rate of glycolysis is more than 200 times higher than that of normal tissue cells. However, the high glycolysis rate of cancer cells does not match the growth and proliferation rate of the cells, for example, the proliferation rate of many normal epithelia of digestive system is much faster than that of cancer cells. Why? The answer lies in the fact that cancer cells have evolved such a high rate of glycolysis, first of all, in order to meet their need for malignant survival against autostabilisis. Only on the premise of anti–autostabilisis, can cancer cells grow and proliferate malignantly. Furthermore, lactic acid production, which cascades with the high consumption of glucose by glycolysis, constitutes another important factor in malignant consumption of cancer cells. Compared with normal cells, the lactate production of cancer cells with malignant biological behaviors is much higher than that of normal cells by two orders of magnitude. In order to avoid accumulative acidosis caused by such a large amount of lactic acid production and to compensate for the consumption of glucose in glycolysis, the body has to metabolize energy through the lactic acid cycle (also known as the Cori cycle, named after Carl Ferdinand Cori, the discoverer of the Cori cycle and the 1947 Nobel Laureate in physiology or medicine). However, this process is also premised on consuming the corresponding ATP. Therefore, under the influence of high energy consumption of high–speed glycolysis of cancer cells, high–load Cori cycle, and high–malignant growth of cancer cells, it is inevitable for the body to become cachexia. Of course, the secondary physiological and biochemical metabolic disorders caused by these high–energy – consumption metabolisms will naturally play a role in "boosting the flames". Therefore, compared with benign tumors weighing tens of kilograms, it is not difficult to understand why small malignant tumors can cause such a serious cachexia in patients. In theory, for a patient with 0.5 kg of tumor that has highly malignant biological behaviors, the daily amount of food needed to reach at least 3–4 times of that (about 5 kg) of normal people can only balance the energy consumption to maintain malignant cancer survival. Otherwise, cancer has to consume tissue to obtain the energy to survive. So don't try to starve cancer cells by limiting dietary intake, because in this way, it's not cancer cells that starve but patients. This also suggests that solving the problem of highly malignant cancer cells in heterogeneous cancers will win valuable time and opportunity for curing cancer.

2.9 Why does heterogeneity make cancer difficult to treat

It is not difficult to understand the heterogeneity of cancer cells by moleculargenetics and MIGI principles. Cancer cells are very different. Various molecular signaling pathways like spider webs form a dazzling "map" of roads leading to "rome": cell's functional goal. Although the current target discovery for various signaling pathways is changing with each passing day, it can never keep up with the star–like variation patterns and speed on the "map". But there is an idiom in China, which is called "all changes are inseparable from their ancestors". It philosophically states that, no matter how the cancer cells change, the outcome of selective adaptation should conform to such a basic and simple truth that they can survive. Therefore, in terms of the survival mode of cancer, its heterogeneity is divided into two simple forms: oxidative phosphorylation or aerobic glycolysis as the main metabolic mode. These two situations can not only encompass the key biological behaviors of cancer cells, but also concisely determine the curable therapeutic regimens solving the difficult treatment problems of most cancers. Because each cancer cell metabolizes differently, after killing the primary chemo–radiotherapy–sensitive cancer cells whose main metabolic mode is aerobic glycolysis, the residual chemo–radiotherapy –tolerant cancer cells close to normal metabolism will become the dominant group and continue to grow. Without understanding this principle, the consequent treatment will be in a "difficult" predicament. If the concept of classifying heterogeneity based on the metabolic patterns is applied to guide the design of clinical therapeutic strategies, the local treatment measures (such as routine or minimally invasive surgery) to reduce the tumor burden can be taken as far as possible to further treat the residual cancers after the BAG therapy. At this time, the cancer will grow in a way close to benign tumors. Under the protection of BAG regimen to prevent and treat cancer metastasis, the eradicative surgery will play its unique therapeutic role.

2.10 Why cancer cells take the aerobic glycolysis route

Normal cells are metabolized by aerobic oxidation (oxidative phosphorylation) under aerobic conditions. Cells that follow thistricarboxylic acid cycle (also known as the Krebs cycle, named after Hans Adolf Krebs, Nobel laureate and discoverer of the cycle) can produce higher ATP output, i. e. 36 molecules of ATP per molecule of glucose consumed. Many cancer cells, even with adequate oxygen supply, still follow a low−productivity metabolic pathway, namely aerobic glycolysis, in which one molecule of glucose produces 2 molecules of ATP only. This is the famous Warburg effect named after Nobel laureate Otto Heinrich Warburg. Why does the Warburg effect occur? Because without the metabolic pathway of the tricarboxylic acid cycle, the key GTP production link will naturally be lost. In addition, the low ATP yield of aerobic glycolysis mode will correspondingly reduce the conversion of ATP to GTP. GTP is an indispensable "building" raw material for the construction of cytoskeleton (microtubules) in large demand. The large reduction of GTP will have an important impact on the assembly of microtubules. Moreover, the decrease of ATP will correspondingly affect the energy consumption required for microtubules to produce compacting force when the cells are rounded. With the decrease of microtubule assembly and nuclear compaction, cancer cells can evade the fatal and senescent fate of circompactosis and MIGI through anti−autostabilisis.

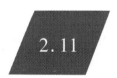

2.11 Why does hypoxia lead to malignant growth and metastasis of cancer cells

The principle is similar to Warburg effect. However, the hypoxia effect is caused by the environment causing anaerobic fermentation, not aerobic glycolysis. No matter what aerobic or anaerobic fermentation, its essence is glycolysis. Hypoxia can change the metabolic mode of cancer cells from aerobic oxidation to anaerobic glycolysis. This metabolic change makes it possible for cancer cells that did not take the aerobic glycolysis pathway to break through the original growth pattern and change from a growth pattern similar to that of benign tumors to a pattern with more malignant biological behaviors. Once anaerobic glycolysis caused by hypoxia falls to the threshold of GTP production, the malignant phenotype driven by environment will be exhibited as caused by aerobic glycolysis, i. e. disordered-growth, invasion and metastasis.

2. 12 Why do cancers have distant metastasis in their "early stages" of their onset

Clinically, many cancers found at the time of initial diagnosis have been metastatic lesions. However, their primary lesions could not be detected by the existing technology. Why does this happen? According to the principle of autostabilisis (circompactosis and lethal MIGI), exfoliated cells can escape the "brake" of autostabilisis as long as mutations of genes or epigenetic changes can lead to metabolic changes, from oxidative phosphorylation to aerobic glycolysis. Once the cancer cells fall off and enter the circulatory system, they may form metastatic foci (of course, adhesion and anchoring conditions may play a supporting role). So in the early stage of cancer metastasis, as long as the mutation of individual cell fulfills the change of metabolic pattern, it can survive in the circulatory system by avoiding the constraints of circompactosis and lethal MIGI, thus leading to distant metastasis. Moreover, the metastasis will show a rapidly growing phenotype of malignancy. At this time, cancer cells in the primary site may die out due to inadaptable selection for survival due to various reasons; they may also grow slowly with a low-grade malignant phenotype (metastatic cancers may have genetic variations different from the primary cancer due to the heterogeneity); or, they may show delayed malignant growth with later genetic mutations and epigenetic changes.

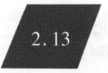

2. 13 Why can one event cause "chromothripsis" of large-scale gene mutations

In 2011, Philip J. and other scientists reported in Cell magazine that by sequencing the DNA of chronic lymphoblastic leukemia, a phenomenon of large-scale gene mutation and chromosome rearrangement caused byone event was discovered and named Chromothripsis. The word Chromothripsis comes from Greek, where Chromo and thripsis refer to "chromosome" and "fragmentation", respectively. The whole word means "chromosome fragmentation", describing the extent to which one event leads to large-scale variation of DNA. This phenomenon has been confirmed in many types of cancers in subsequent studies. Although the mechanism behind this phenomenon is unknown, the revealing of this phenomenon itself is a revolutionary discovery.

For a long time, it has been believed that the carcinogenesis of cells is due to the accumulation of long-term gene mutations. This discovery of Chromothripsis overturns the traditional understanding of carcinogenesis. Aguilera A. et al. published a review in the Annual Review of Genetics in 2013 that "Understanding the molecular basis of chromothripsis will certainly shed light on our knowledge of genome instability and its consequences." and that "it is too early to know the causes of this phenomenon". With the extensive development of recent research, several models have emerged to explain the mechanism of chromothripsis, including nucleosome model, ionizing radiation during mitosis, abortion of apoptosis and telomere dysfunction. However, in terms of genomic instability caused by cell rounding, the most universal and inevitable biological event in advanced multicellular living beings, as well as the principle and confirmatory experiments that cell rounding can cause large-scale catastrophic changes at the genetic and chromosomal levels, MIGI can undoubtedly provide us with detailed clues to understand, explain and elucidate the mechanism of Chromothripsis.

2. 14　Why do adolescent osteosarcoma patients often have a history of trauma

Adolescent osteosarcoma is a bone cancer with high malignancy and mortality. Long-term clinical data show that adolescent osteosarcoma patients often have a history of trauma. Due to the lack of understanding of the causal relationship between physical trauma and bone cancer with genetic variation, whether trauma is an inducer of bone cancer has become a long-standing controversialissue. With the development of research, new data provide a basis for clarifying the relationship between trauma and the incidence of bone cancer in adolescents. Genetically, about 33% of bone cancers have chromothripsis. This is in good agreement with the clinical data about 1/3 (33%) of adolescent osteosarcoma patients with traumatic history. Is there a causal relationship between the bone cancer and Chromothripsis? MIGI can provide clues to explain their causality. The main characteristic of trauma is inflammation caused by physical factors. Inflammation caused by any factor can destroy the local tissue structure. The destruction of tissue microenvironment will affect the connection of cell-to-cell and cell-to-adjacent-tissues, resulting in cell rounding and re-spreading. Teenagers are in the stage of skeletal growth and development, and the cells associated with skeletal growth are in an active state of proliferation. At this time, the cell rounding and re-spreading of proliferation cells will naturally lead to the occurrence of MIGI. MIGI is just the basis of the formation of Chromothripsis. So theoretically, there is a close relationship between trauma and adolescent bone cancer. Bone cancer is a malignant tumor with high incidence in adolescents, which seriously threatens the life and health of adolescents. Understanding the pathogenesis of adolescent bone cancer has important clinical significance in preventing and treating this disease.

2.15 Is hayflick limit caused by telomere shortening

In 1961, LeonardHayflick, an American anatomist, discovered that when human normal fibroblasts were cultured in vitro, they stopped dividing after 40 to 60 population doublings (PDs). Later, this phenomenon was called the Hayflick limit, and became a well-known classical hypothesis to explain the life limit of normal cells. However, there was no basis for explaining the mechanism of this phenomenon until 2009, when the Nobel Prize in Physiology or Medicine was awarded for discovering the mechanism of protecting chromosomes by telomeres and telomerase. From then on, people began to use it to explain the supporting mechanism behind the Hayflick limit phenomenon. That is, every time a normal somatic cell undergoes chromosomal replication and mitosis, the telomere length will be shortened to a certain extent. When the telomere is shortened to a threshold of length (there is no accurate numerical report yet), the cell will stop dividing, so the telomere length is also called the "clock of life". However, scientists have also found a problem that normal fibroblasts of mice retain longer telomeres and highly active telomerase (an enzyme that maintain telomere length) after 20−30 PD cycles, but they also stop mitosis and die as normal fibroblasts of human beings. Why? People can't explain it. Jack Szostak, one of the winners of the 2009 Nobel Prize in Physiology or Medicine for discovering telomere protection mechanisms, called it a good puzzle. In such a case, some scientists have helplessly explained that mouse cells may be different from human cells. Is that true? If you have done cell culture, you will know that there is such a seemingly ordinary process in cell culture, and it has to be used as a routine cell processing step — passage. Usually, the process of passage of adherent cultured cells is that when the cultured cells are spread and confluent in the culture vessel, they are stripped off from the culture vessel wall by some means (such as the most common and classical treatment—digestion with trypsin or mechanical scraping) to form dispersed single cell suspension or small pieces, and then the passaged cells are re−implanted according to different experimental purposes. The problem then arises. Once the cell is peeled off, its stress state changes immediately. The cells present rounding because of both the sharp decrease of pulling force, produced by the actin filaments anchored in the extracellular matrix and/or connected to the cell−to−cell junctions, and the hydromechanical effect. The nucleus is consequently compacted violently by the compacting force produced by the microtubules. At this time, the cells face two fates. One is that if the cells can not get spreading in time, the death of suspension cells, i. e. circompactosis, will be caused by the effects of nuclear compaction, i. e. restriction of RNA transcription, inability to translate proteins, degradation of existing RNA, inactivation of enzymes and disorder of biochemical reactions. The second fate is that even if the cells can get spreading in time, the dissociation of single-stranded DNA-binding proteins such as RPA and POT1 from their bound single-stranded DNA, which is caused by nuclear compaction, will results in the loss of protection of 80,000 to 160,000 single-stranded DNA chains at replication forks and single-stranded DNA chains at telomeres in each cell at the stage of DNA synthesis. The consequence is that single-stranded DNA binding proteins lose their important functions in preventing the formation of incorrect secondary DNA structures and avoiding telomere end fusion. In other words, under the intense compaction of nuclear space, a large number of unprotected single-stranded DNA sequences are exposed to each other that can produce non-physiological sticky pairings and interact with each other. This will drastically increase the chances of incorrect intra-strand, inter-strand, intra-chromosome and inter-chromosome base pairing, forming DNA secondary structure and chromosome end fusion. It will inevitably result in microtubule-induced genomic instability (MIGI), large-scale gene mutations and chromosomal aberrations. Indeed, our experimental results demonstrated that abnormal karyotype formation was detected in human fibroblasts after three times of cell rounding (Figure 2-3). In addition, when the cells underwent about 50 times of cell rounding (highly consistent with Hayflick's population doubling and passage times) but not 50 times of population doublings, and only cultured for about 0. 8 months (6. 25-7. 5 times shorter than Hayflick's 5-6 months), the cells lost the ability to make population doubling and stepped into senescence and death. The experimental results of cultured cells that underwent two times of cell-rounding/one day (i. e. six times of cell-rounding/3 days/ 1PD) suggested that MIGI was the main cause of Hayflick limit, not telomere shortening. Because the actual times of population doublings of the experimental cells differ greatly from the population doubling times of Hayflick limit, which is totally inconsistent with the hypothesis. Moreover, the author has done a very interesting experiment. Normal human fibroblasts were cultured under conventional conditions, but the only way of passage was to use the author invented "cell membrane creeping in" technique which could avoid the rounding of passaged cells. At the end of the continuous experiment for 10 months, the cells cultured by this method experienced more than 100 PD, but did not show the senescence and death phenomenon as the conventional cell subculture. This further suggests that Hayflick limit is only an artificial phenomenon and result caused by cell-rounding in vitro, which can not reflect the physiological state of cells in vivo, nor can it be used as a classical index to explain the aging and life-span of normal cells. However, the deduction of Hayflick limit's cell culture method, as a well-recognized and classically mature repeatable experiment, can provide a typical example of the important role of MIGI.

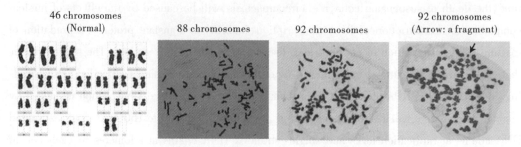

Figure 2-3　Abnormal karyotypes of normal human fibroblasts caused by cell rounding

2. 16　What is the role of "junk" DNA, is "junk" DNA real junk

On the 125th anniversary of the publication of Science magazine in 2005, a major scientific question "What is all that'junk' doing in our genomes? " was published. For a long time, there has been a great controversy in academic field about whether "junk" DNA is junk or not. Because, with the progress of research-in-depth, it has been found that some "junk" DNA may be involved in the regulation of individual genes, nevertheless, there is still a large number of "junk" DNA, especially a large number of simple repetitive sequences in "junk" DNA, which can not be verified for its function, so it is still considered as "junk". However, the author of this paper finds that the so-called "junk" DNA is not "junk" by any means, and it has unique indispensability in the aspect of autostabilisis. That is to say, without "junk" DNA, it is impossible for advanced living beings to achieve autostabilisis. Why? The reason is cell exfoliation is a natural property of advanced multicellular living beings. Therefore, in order to prevent cell in situ disordered growth and heterotopic implantation, and thus achieve autostabilisis, the body has evolved three key factors for this machinery: one is the compacting force that can make the nucleus compacted; the other is the changeable cellular space where the physiological activities of the nucleus can be carried out and the nuclear compaction can be achieved due to pathological cell-rounding; and the third is the so-called "junk" DNA. When cells are pathologically rounded, only through the compacting force produced by microtubules can the nuclear space be compacted drastically, so that genomic DNA loses the nuclear space needed for RNA transcription and DNA replication, and can the "brake" type of autostabilisis formed by circompactosis and lethal MIGI be realized. In the process of autostabilisis, "junk" DNA plays an important role as a "brake pad". Because the nuclear membrane and DNA double helix are rigid solid structures, the nucleus will be compacted by deformation caused by the pressure of rigid microtubules' "sliding" when the cell is rounded, rather than the elastic contraction of the nucleus itself. Therefore, the size of the nucleus under physiological conditions plays a decisive role in the magnitude of the force required for compressive deformation and compaction. If the genome removes 98.5% of the "junk" DNA, the cell rounding should correspond to two theoretically hypothetical compaction–models: ① the nucleus is compacted according to the true size. At this time, only 1.5% of the DNA density of the original genome can not lead to the formation of nuclear–compaction space that restricts RNA transcription and DNA replication, so circompactosis and lethal MIGI can not be achieved. ② If the initial nucleus size is 1.5% of the normal nucleus, it is impossible for the nucleus to complete the compaction at the compaction–ratio of the true cell rounding, because in this case, only the rigid space–occupancy of the nuclear–solid components, such as the nuclear membrane and nuclear skeleton, and the force produced by the microtubules per unit area and volume at the end of the compacting process as well as the deformable physical–condition of the nucleus by force, form the restrictive factors that make the compaction impossible. In addition, the reduction of genomic DNA to 1.5% not only means that the density of DNA decreases greatly, but also the entanglement of DNA strands decreases drastically. Therefore, in theory, to achieve the "brake" effect of RNA transcription and DNA replication in this case, the nuclear compaction–ratio has to be much larger than the true compaction–ratio. Furthermore, when genomic DNA is reduced to 1.5% of the true DNA, in theory, the modes of forming chromosome, spindle, mitosis and inheritance, which the advanced multicellular living beings evolved in order to form differentiated cells, functionalized tissues and organs, should no longer exist. The way of inheritance, growth and proliferation should be similar to that of protozoa. In a word, "junk" DNA plays an essential role in the establishment and evolution of the autostabilic machinery of advanced multicellular living beings, which is fundamental and indispensable for the space–occupancy effect.

2.17 Why can chemotherapy lead to metastasis of cancer cells

Metastasis is an important cause of death in more than 90% of cancer patients. Traditionally, chemotherapy has been considered as a treatment to prevent cancer metastasis. However, recently with the researches–in–depth, people began to pay attention to the problem of cancer metastasis caused by chemotherapy. Because traditional chemotherapy lacks specific inhibitors for cancer metastasis, the microenvironment-damage caused by chemotherapy can lead to cancer cells' rounding, MIGI, gene mutation, metabolic aerobic-glycolysis transformation, and its ultimate anti-circompactosis cascade events. Moreover, non-lethal doses of drugs (such as vinblastine and taxanes) that interfere with microtubule assembly of cancer cells can produce anti-circompactosis effects similar to that of aerobic glycolysis, which constitute the preconditions of cancer metastasis for breaching the autostabilisis. Furthermore, the destruction of the microenvironment of cancer tissue caused by chemotherapeutics will make it easier for cancer cells to enter the circulatory system, which undoubtedly creates a convenient condition for cancer cell's metastasis. In addition, acquired or induced drug resistance of cancer cells to chemotherapy can lead to cell-heterogeneity-remodeling with drug-resistance-priority in cancer tissues, which makes the metastasizing and metastasized cancer cells have greater drug resistance. These results suggest that in the absence of specific inhibitory intervention on metastatic cancer cells, any damage to the microenvironment of cancer tissues, tissue repair inhibition, inflammation caused by various causes, as well as the drugs interfering with microtubule assembly can lead to metastasis of cancer cells. Therefore, specific treatment for cancer metastasis is the most important part of cancer therapy.

2.18 Why can statins cause rhabdomyolysis

Statins have beenworldwidely used as effective lipid-lowering drugs. However, the relationship between statins and rhabdomyolysis is a key point for attention in the clinical application of statins. Why? Because striated muscle is the type of tissue that constitutes the skeletal muscle in various human motion systems, and rhabdomyolysis can cause serious consequences. The movement of skeletal muscles depends on the supply of a large amount of energy. Under normal oxygen supply and daily physiological activities, the rhabdomyus produces ATP in the form of oxidative phosphorylation mainly through the tricarboxylic acid cycle (TCA) to provide energy for the activities. Its oxidative metabolites are mainly CO_2 and water. However, in the case of local or systemic hypoxia caused by various oxygen insufficiency factors and long-term and large-amount exercise, the rhabdomyus will open the metabolic pathway of glycolysis because of lack of oxygen or energy supply. Although the rate of energy-production of glycolysis is faster than that of aerobic oxidation, yet the productivity of glycolysis is much lower than that of aerobic oxidation (2 ATP : 36 ATP). Only through a large amount of glycolysis metabolism can compensatory energy be provided. However, a large amount of energy-production of glycolysis process has to produce a large number of metabolites lactic acid. The accumulation of a large amount of lactic acid in skeletal muscle cells can lead to the destruction of cell biochemical function. Serious accumulation of lactic acid can lead to catastrophic cell toxicity and death. Because the rhabdomyus itself can not use lactic acid, only lactic acid cycle (also known as Cori cycle, named after Carl Ferdinand Cori and his wife, the winner of the 1947 Nobel Prize in Physiology or Medicine) becomes the main way to drain lactic acid into the blood and recycle it through the liver to synthesize glucose. Monocarboxylate transporter 4 (MCT4) plays a key role in the process of lactic acid excretion from striated muscle, which is responsible for transporting intracellular lactic acid to extracellular sites. Once the lactic acid efflux of MCT4 is blocked, the lactic acid in the cells will be accumulated, and the consequences are catastrophic. However, statins are the blockers of MCT4, so it is not difficult to understand why the side effects of statins can cause rhabdomyolysis. This suggests that people should avoid hypoxia and excessive exercise caused by various reasons during the course of taking statins. Especially for patients who are seriously ill in bed, attention should be paid to the prevention of circulatory ischemia and hypoxia caused by local compression and restraint.

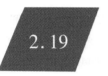

2.19 Why do the cells of advanced multicellular living beings have nuclei

The intrinsic characteristic of advanced multicellularliving beings is the establishment of tissue-and-organ structure, which is the basis of maintaining advanced multicellular biological functions. In order to complete the metabolism of tissues and organs, repair the damage caused by various unavoidable damage factors in the process of life, and maintain the normal physiological structure of tissues, the body has evolved the autostabilic machinery composed of circompactosis and lethal MIGI as the core mechanisms to prevent abnormal proliferation and growth of cells. The nuclei, microtubules, mitochondria and Junk DNA are the four core structural elements of the autostabilic machinery. It is just because of the synergistic effect of these four unique cell core structural elements that advanced multicellular living beings can establish the autostabilisis of the cells. Furthermore, it is with the autostabilic machinery that the normal tissue structure can be maintained and the immune defense system against abnormal immunogen can be established. Only then can the organisms guarantee their reproduction.

2.20 What is the relationship among mechanical force and cell proliferation and tumorigenesis

Active cell proliferation coupled with corresponding mutations in cancer suppressor and oncogene constitutes the basis of cancer occurrence. It can be said that there is no cancer without proliferation, because proliferation plays a key role in the process of carcinogenesis from two aspects. One is that proliferation increases the occurrence of MIGI, that is, proliferative cells can create conditions for large-scale gene mutations and evolutionary selection of cancer. The other is that only through proliferation can the genetic fixation of mutations in cancer-related genes and the formation and growth of cancer tissues be completed. The effect of mechanical tension can stimulate the active proliferation of cells by removing the restriction of nuclear space of DNA activity produced by cell density and enhancing the accessibility of growth factors caused by basement membrane tension. For example, surgical skin expansion for repairing injuries, surgical limb lengthening, and extruded epithelial hyperplasia and keratinization (commonly known as callus) are due to this cellular-and-molecular biological role. Moreover, under the action of mechanical tension on the cells of organs and tissues, the event of cell rounding caused by various inflammations lays a foundation for the evolutionary selection of carcinogenic gene mutations caused by MIGI, which makes the carcinogenesis easier to occur. Therefore, appropriate measures should be taken to avoid or eliminate the expanding-tension factors that cause organs to exceed the physiological expansion (such as abnormal gas production of digestive system and food residues caused by unreasonable diet and other factors, as well as poor excretion of feces, and fluid retention in urinary system). These measures have important clinical significance for the prevention of cancer.

2.21 Why are there big differences in the size of various multicellular living bings' bodies and small differences in the size of somatic cells

Nature's creatures are as big as whales and elephants, as small as rats and fleas. Although individual size varies greatly, the difference in somatic cell size is very small. Why? There have been various explanations for the answer to this question, but the vital importance of the "autostabilisis" of advanced multicellular living beings is indispensable. As mentioned earlier, the size of the nucleus is crucial to the survival of cells, and the mechanical structure and stress state of cells are important factors to determine the size of the nucleus. The effect of the compacting force produced by cell rounding on the nucleus is manifested by the compaction of the necessary functional space of DNA in RNA transcription and DNA replication so as to prevent the catastrophic events of abnormally cellular proliferation and growth that can kill the body, in the way like "braking" by circompactosis and lethal MIGI. Whether advanced multicellular beings can realize this "autostabilic" function is determined by the cascade effect of DNA molecular size of cell genome as the key factor. According to this core factor, the appropriate size and proportion of cellular nucleus and cellular volume were optimized. Any change that violates this rule will bring disastrous results to the survival of the organism. Because if the cell nucleus becomes smaller, the physiological activity space of genomic DNA will not be fulfilled. on the contrary, if the cell nucleus becomes larger, a series of factors matching it have to change in violation of natural law. Assuming that the nucleus is a sphere, if its axis diameter is doubled, the DNA size of the cell genome needs to be increased to 8 times the original size to match it. This means that a series of factors such as the molecular weight of "junk" DNA, the number of gene copies, cell volume and cytoskeleton molecules should be increased accordingly. In this case, a lot of biological events of forming the basis of advanced living beings, such as the formation of the circulatory system, the tissues, the organs, the mode of energy supply, the mechanism of minimizing the risk of cell stress damage, the mechanism of minimizing the influence of body movement on tissue and cell tension (the dispersion and sharing of force by cell number per unit volume), the mechanism of tissue renewal, and the mechanism of tissue – damage repair, will become impossible. Fortunately, none of this can be true. Otherwise, advanced multicellular living beings cannot be produced. Therefore, although individual sizes vary greatly, it is just because the nature optimizes the cellular and nuclear sizes of advanced multicellular living beings to form the autostabilic machinery with the four key structural elements of mitochondria, microtubules, nuclei and "junk" DNA that advanced multicellular living beings with various body sizes can come into the world.

2.22   Why do mitochondria have their own DNA and genetic system

Cells need energy to maintain their life activities. Mitochondria are energy factories ofthe cells in advanced multicellular living beings. Normal energy supply of normal cells mainly comes from oxidative phosphorylation in mitochondria. Thus, mitochondria are essential for cell survival. However, all the activities of mitochondria as organelles in cells, including their own duplication and renewal, as well as their energy-productivity process, are catalyzed by enzymatic reactions. The main component of the enzyme is protein. Although most of the enzymes and proteins involved in biochemical reactions in cells and the proteins that make up organelles are encoded by nuclear DNA, the genome of mitochondrion's own genetic system directly encodes its unique enzymes and protein products, which are closely related to oxidative phosphorylation to produce ATP. Generally speaking, enzymatic proteins belong to short-lived proteins. Therefore, in order to complete their updating, it is necessary to be able to timely transcribe RNA from their encoded DNA. However, when cells are in M phase of cell cycle or rounded due to various reasons, DNA in the nucleus is in a compacted state, and their physiological RNA transcription activity will be limited, while cells still need energy supply at this time. In this case, if mitochondria do not have their own DNA and genetic system, the consequences will be unimaginable.

2.23 How do retroviruses mutate through host cells

Retroviruses are RNA viruses with high mutation rates. For replication, the virus can utilize the reverse transcriptase of the virus itself to synthesize DNA by using viral RNA as template. Then the virus DNA is integrated into the genome of the host cell. The replication process of the virus is accomplished by the replication system of host cell. Since the genetic information of the virus is integrated into the genome of the host cell, it means that the MIGI effect affecting the host cell may also affect the genomic DNA encoding the virus's inheritance (Figure 2-4). Moreover, inflammation can cause MIGI events, and viral infection itself is an inflammatory factor. Therefore, this will increase the incidence of MIGI and the viral variation. However, the genome of the virus is small, and severe mutations may be lethal and invalid mutations, which may be a limiting factor for the viral variation.

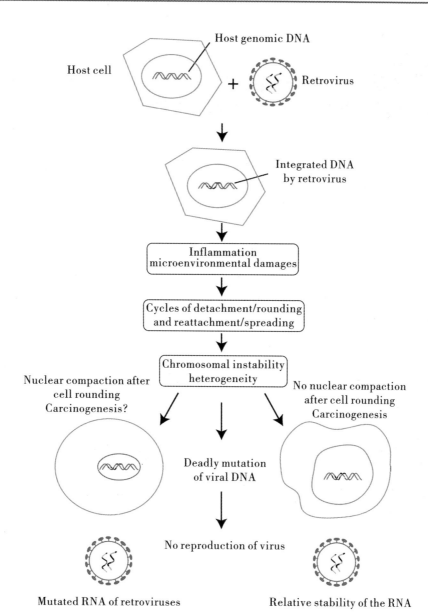

Figure 2-4   Schematic diagram of the theory of retrovirus gene mutation

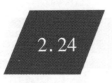

How can embryonic stem cells be removed from mixed cells for therapeutic research

2. 24

As stem cell research has shifted from the initial discovery study to the currently eagerly anticipated application study, it has been realized that there is a great risk of generating malignant tumors by implanting undifferentiated embryonic stem cells (including induced pluripotent stem cells) in vivo. Therefore, the focus of research has shifted to the induced differentiation of embryonic stem cells. However, stem cell therapy requires a large number of cells. How to isolate and purify differentiated cells from a large number of mixed population of embryonic stem cells and differentiated cells, that is, to remove undifferentiated embryonic cells from the mixed population, is a huge bottleneck challenge. Now, according to the metabolic characteristics of the aerobic glycolysis of embryonic stem cells, a solution to remove embryonic stem cells from mixed cells based on the principles of simplicity, economy, efficiency and safety can be provided by using a drug treatment strategy similar to that described in this paper.

Does intervention of metabolic pattern of glycolysis have impact on blastomere embryonic stem cells in early pregnancy

2. 25

Embryonic stem cells are undifferentiated cells of early embryos formed by the growth, division and proliferation of fertilized eggs. Its metabolic characteristics are mainly aerobic glycolysis. In theory, the drugs that inhibit lactic acid excretion channels (including statins and proton pump inhibitors) can affect the survival and growth of embryonic stem cells at the stage when embryonic stem cells have not yet grown and differentiated into committed stem cells. Therefore, whether this interventional therapy has the efficacy of contraceptives in terminating pregnancy and harmful effects on embryonic development needs further study.

2.26   What is the mechanism of plant protoplast asexual breeding

Plant protoplast asexual breeding is an important breeding method without exogenous gene transfer. Compared with the methods of radiation breeding and spaceborne breeding, plant protoplast asexual breeding has the characteristics of economy, safety, easy realization and can be used for a wide range of research purposes. Now, it has been widely used in crop breeding, flower breeding and other aspects. Unfortunately, the mechanism behind plant protoplast asexual breeding has not yet been elucidated, although more than half a century of research has passed since the initial acquisition of protoplasts. Undoubtedly, it is of great significance for the development of plant breeding technology to clarify its mechanism. Through the analysis of the operation steps and results of plant protoplast asexual breeding, we can clearly find the core rule of this technology – cell rounding, and once the cell is rounded, it will inevitably lead to the occurrence of MIGI. This is precisely why the genetic traits of plant protoplast will change after protoplast isolation and culture, and this change is uncontrollable.

References

[1] GUO Q,LIAO X L,WANG X W,et al. Cell rounding cause genomic instability by dissociation of single-stranded DNA-binding proteins [DB/OL]. bioRxiv doi:https://doi.org/10.1101/463653.2018.

[2] FRISCH S M,FRANCIS H. Disruption of epithelial cell-matrix interactions induces apoptosis [J]. J Cell Biol,1994,124(4): 619-626.

[3] CHEN C S,MRKSICH M,HUANG S,et al. Geometric control of cell life and death [J]. Science,1997,276(5317): 1425-1428.

[4] GUO Q,TANG W,KOKUDO N,et al. Epidermal growth factor-mediated growth control of confluent mammary epithelial cells cultured on artificial basement membrane [J]. Int J Mol Med,2005,16(3): 395-399.

[5] YAO N Y,O'DONNELL M. SnapShot:The replisome [J]. Cell,2010,141(6):1088-1088.

[6] CREAGER R L,LI Y,MACALPINE D M. SnapShot: Origins of DNA replication [J]. Cell,2015,161(2): 418.

[7] WANG K R,XUE S B,LIU H T. Cell biology [M]. Beijing:Beijing Normal University Press,1990.

[8] MARINO N,NAKAYAMA J,COLLINS J W,et al. Insights into the biology and prevention of tumor metastasis provided by the Nm23 metastasis suppressor gene [J]. Cancer Metastasis Rev,2012,31(3-4): 593-603.

[9] SHASHNI B,SHARMA K,SINGH R,et al. Coffee component hydroxyl hydroquinone (HHQ) as a putative ligand for PPAR gamma and implications in breast cancer [J]. BMC Genomics,2013,14 (Suppl 5):1-16.

[10] PINHEIRO C,LONGATTO-FILHO A,AZEVEDO-SILVA J,et al. Role of monocarboxylate transporters in human cancers: state of the art [J]. Bioenerg. Biomembr,2012,44 (1):127-139.

[11] WARBURG O,POSENER K,NEGELEIN E. Über den Stoffwechsel der Carcinomzelle [J]. Biochem Zeitschr,1925,4(12):309-344.

[12] SKLOOT R. The immortal life of henrietta lacks [M]. New York: Crown/Random House, 2010.

[13] AGUILERA A,GARCíA-MUSE T. Causes of genome instability [J]. Annu Rev Genet, 2013,117(1):1-32.

[14] KANSARA M,TENG M W,SMYTH M J,et al. Translational biology of osteosarcoma

[J]. Nat Rev Cancer,2014,14(11):722-735.

[15] YANG J Y,CHENG F W,WONG K C,et al. Initial presentation and management of osteosarcoma,and its impact on disease outcome [J]. Hong Kong Med J 2009,15(6):434-439.

[16] SHAMIR M,BAR-ON Y,PHILLIPS R,et al. SnapShot: Timescales in cell biology [J]. Cell,2016,164(6):1302-1302.